A Caregiver's Journey

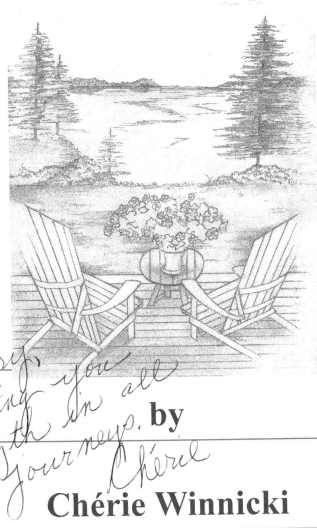

Marie,
Wishing you
strength in all
your Journeys. **by**
Chérie

Chérie Winnicki

Text ©2013 Chérie Winnicki

Illustration ©2013 Phil Reynolds

Design ©2013 Laurie Barrows
"Making the World a Happier Place,
One Smile at a Time" ™
www.LaurieBarrows.com

Copy Editor:Amy Johnson

Published by Tiger Mountain Books
Contact Kathie Horsman
Kathie@tigermountainbooks.com

ISBN-13: 978-1493536832
ISBN: 1493536834

Printed in the United States of America

Published in the United States of America

There are only four kinds of people in this world:

those who have been caregivers,

those who are currently caregivers,

those who will be caregivers,

and those who will need caregivers.

Rosalynn Carter

Helping Yourself Help Others

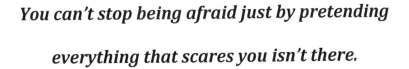

You can't stop being afraid just by pretending

everything that scares you isn't there.

Michael Marshall

The Upright Man

1. The Phone Call

The phone call came late on a crisp, fall evening. I knew when I answered and it was the doctor asking to talk to Bob that something was wrong.

We had retired a year or so earlier from the East Coast and settled near the Rocky Mountains. After living so many years away from family, we decided to make the leap and move closer to them. We knew we would enjoy the great outdoors in Colorado with all the hiking, biking, and tennis for which the area was known.

Bob had decided that he wanted to retire early. He was feeling the stress of his job more and more and was just plain tired. He was only fifty-eight years old. It seemed young to pack it up and walk away from his career as an engineer and program manager. He just did not have the energy to keep up with everything and blamed his exhaustion on job-related stress.

I wasn't ready to retire from my teaching career. I was rejuvenated after taking years off to be a stay-at-home mom. Going back to teaching was like starting over, but with a new level of energy, patience, and wisdom. I was able to dedicate more time to my students since my own children were growing up and very independent.

Bob traveled frequently for business, and there were long evenings alone filled with correcting papers and preparing lesson plans. With no one home, it was wonderful having a purpose and knowing I was making a difference in the lives of the students. I was exhausted most of the time, but the feeling of knowing I was making a difference outweighed being tired.

So when Bob came home one day and said he wanted to retire, I had mixed emotions. We knew when retirement came we were escaping the winters of the East Coast. We hadn't narrowed in on any special place, but we knew it meant a move. As with all decisions, we sat with our lists and compared pros and cons of various areas.

The Rocky Mountains won because of family being there. We looked at it as another adventure in our lives, and we would go forward with no looking back. I wasn't ready to say goodbye to teaching. I could feel it in my bones that I was doing something worthy and productive. I loved the interaction and the many success stories of student after student accomplishing their goals.

The decision was made to retire. After committing, I discovered that leaving teaching at that time was one year short of a mandatory requirement. If I left, I would not be able to receive any health care benefits. Should I stay and teach one more year, on my own? Should I go and forget the benefits? It was a difficult decision. I knew in my heart I was not going to live a year away from Bob. We went forward and made the move.

My last gift to the senior class was being the speaker for their graduation. I spoke of journeys: past, present, and future. I compared their new adventure to mine. How we were similar with having unknowns ahead of us. I encouraged them to look at the journey as an adventure. My advice was to live it with spirit and enthusiasm and face the unknown head-on. Little did I know what that journey was going to be for me.

Our first year of retirement was full of adjustments. Moving close to family after being away from them for thirty years took time to adjust. My expectations of joining this circle of love was met with the reality that the circle was more like a big pot with each member taking turns stirring the pot.

Bob and I had to adjust to being together 24-7. After years of independent jobs and activities we were in each other's paths all day long. He wanted to direct me to projects, and I had my own ideas and lists of activities. He went to the gym regularly, took walks, and read, but he wanted me to spend my time doing these activities with him.

I felt smothered. I took on teaching a class at a local community college. Thrown into the mix was planning a wedding for our daughter, Anastasia, to be held the summer after our first year of retirement.

Yet another thing added spice to this long list of adjustments. There had been a big special report on the news warning women who had been taking Prempro for menopause. The news indicated it could be harmful taken for a long period of time. Acting on my own instinct, I went off it—cold turkey. I went through severe emotional ups and downs for months. I am surprised we survived that first year of retirement.

Anastasia's wedding was held in late summer up in the mountains. Bob and I decided to take a short road trip to help recoup from the year of wedding planning and spending. We drove to Santa Fe and just enjoyed the quiet time together. The travel was tiring for Bob. We discussed his need to see the doctor once we got home.

There were many theories of what could be causing his tiredness. The obvious one, living at a higher elevation, made sense. We had moved from sea level to settle at a mile high. Bob was concerned about the cause, but really just wanted to get back to enjoying his exercise and daily life. His attitude was, "Let's find out what is wrong and fix it." The doctors decided after months of extensive tests trying to discover why he was tired that he should have a bone marrow biopsy.

The phone call came from the doctor giving Bob the results of his bone barrow biopsy. The words, **myelodysplastic syndrome**, meant nothing to Bob. His first question to the doctor was, "Is it CANCER?" The answer was not a clear yes or no. The doctor said that statistically he had three to five years to live. He was told to make an appointment to come into the office and discuss the results. He hung up and just stared at me. Three to five years to live. That is all he had heard. He went white.

The next few days we spent much time surfing the net for facts about myelodysplastic syndrome, or MDS (www.mds-foundation.org). We learned much about the disease.

- There is no cure for MDS.
- Survival of MDS is only possible through a high-risk bone marrow transplant.
- It is a disease that affects the bone marrow and blood.
- Some types of MDS are mild and easily managed, while other types are severe and life-threatening.
- It can develop into a fast-growing, severe leukemia.
- About 10,000 to 15,000 people in the U.S. are diagnosed every year with MDS.
- The bone marrow does not make enough normal blood cells for the body with MDS.
- The cause of MDS is most often unknown. Some people with MDS might be linked to heavy exposure to some chemicals, such as petroleum and certain solvents, or to radiation and chemotherapy.

We walked into the meeting with the doctor with many questions. What caused this? What did he do that he should not have? Did fertilizing the lawn all those years cause this? Did he expose himself at work to some chemical? The search was on to discover a reason for his diagnosis.

... I did it my way.

Frank Sinatra
My Way

2. Searching for Answers

The doctor's visit was very somber. We just weren't at the place to see anything positive concerning Bob having MDS. I remember looking around at the people in the waiting room and thinking how depressing it was to see all the sick people. The tears burned my eyes as I realized that we were part of the people in the waiting room, too. After all, we were on the Oncology floor. Cancer. The unknown was so hard to handle. We hoped the doctor would give us some kind of encouragement.

As we sat and listened to the information about the disease, we both were familiar with the words and terms used. We had run into them during our internet searches. Bob wanted to get to the reasons why. He had so many questions to ask. I sat with my paper and pen ready to jot notes. Bob sat with his list of questions. He didn't receive many answers that day.

There really weren't many the doctor could give. His tiredness was due to low counts in his red blood cells. Red blood cells give oxygen to the vital parts of the body. He was warned that his numbers would drop to the point that he would need blood transfusions in order to be strong enough to accomplish daily activities. Once in the car I asked Bob what information he was glad to have. He responded with two positives. Some patients survive up to ten years with this disease. Only his red blood cells were affected, not his white blood cells and platelets.

Each day I watched Bob become more quiet and withdrawn. The teacher in me immediately started organizing all the information we had received from the doctor plus what we had printed off the internet. I found a three-ring binder and started filling it. With a bright yellow marker in my hand, I started highlighting words and paragraphs that I thought noteworthy. Before I knew it, I had one binder full and another one started. I would sit at the counter in the kitchen with a cup of coffee and read. I was insatiable.

All the time I was processing the MDS news by delving into information, Bob drifted further and further into depression and sadness. At that time I really felt I could cheer him up by being lighthearted and tell him news of Anastasia or our son, Robert.

I had always been a fixer and a peacemaker. I tried as a youngster to please and make people happy. My sense of humor had evolved from liking to make people happy. When Anastasia and Robert were young and there were arguments between them I would negotiate an agreeable solution. Even with our children being young adults and living independently, I found myself indulging and spoiling them.

Anastasia loved it, and Robert wished I would let go. As an adult he once said to me, "You were like a helicopter while we were growing up." He made the sound of the blades rotating--blummp-blummp, blummp-blummp. I had to smile while visualizing that. He was so right on in describing me that way. I knew I needed to let go of being the helicopter.

Bob had always been a quiet person. He held things in and processed them privately by pondering about them, including finances, disagreements between us, comparison shopping, and work issues he dealt with before retirement. I never knew his thoughts until they just came out, like when he told me he wanted to retire.

I had no idea he had been thinking about it for a long time. I know it might seem strange to be together in the same house, sit across from each other at the dinner table, and not know what was going on inside his head. At the time it was our pattern, and it had been for thirty years, so dealing with our new crisis meant using the tools we knew and helped us feel comfortable.

One day Bob raised his voice and yelled, "I don't want to read or hear about the information in the binders!" That was it! He said I could make as many folders as I wanted if it helped me feel better, but he did not want to read anything else about MDS. He didn't want me to pass on any tidbits of information. He wanted no more talking about it and for me please to keep it to myself.

At first, my eyes filled with tears as I took his anger personally. For some reason I really heard his words and just went over and sat across from him on the ottoman and said, "I am so sorry. I can't imagine how hard this is for you. I am sorry I have not been more sensitive to you and your feelings."

It broke the silence and the words and tears just came out. He was scared, sad, and depressed. He shared that he really wanted as much information he could get, but that making a binder was not his way.

He said he had been looking into a national conference held annually by an organization called Aplastic Anemia & MDS International Foundation (www.aamds.org). It was having a patient and family conference in Baltimore, Maryland, and he really wanted to attend. We hugged and cried for some time. It was the beginning of our life-changing journey.

Knowledge is of two kinds.
We know a subject ourselves,
or we know where we can find information upon it.

Samuel Johnson

3. Road Trip

The AA&MDSIF Conference was set for the first week of December in Baltimore, MD. We made our reservations for the hotel and attendance at the conference. We had a mission. We were doing SOMETHING. We thought it was all about collecting information from the guest speakers and asking questions and maybe even getting some answers. We were hopeful for the first time since the phone call.

Bob and I had always enjoyed road trips. Other than the obvious reason of seeing the country, it was an opportunity for us to be together and just share the time and space, as we listened to music or books on tapes, talked, or just felt the special time together.

The trip was cross country with many days on the road. We planned enough time to stop and visit friends, Rita and Dan, from our old hometown. Our plans were to continue on to spend Thanksgiving with Anastasia and new husband, Daryl. They had been married only a few months, and it was their first Thanksgiving together.

The saying you can't go back is so true. Visiting our friends and stopping in at the high school where I taught was a wakeup call for me. I look back at my inner conflict during the visit and realize that the awkwardness and the feeling of being out of it that I experienced was really just my own perception. It wasn't that anyone was rude or mean to me. It was that their lives were continuing on, without me in it, and yes, they were doing just fine without my input and ideas.

It was my aha moment. Rita and Dan were going on with life and surviving without our weekly dinners and get-togethers. As they listened to Bob tell them facts about MDS, I realized that trying to describe how we felt about the MDS diagnosis only produced a blur in their eyes. They heard the words, but the fear and anxiety in our souls were uniquely ours.

As we continued on the road trip, our conversation spilled over to our children, Anastasia and Robert, and how they were accepting the news of their dad having a terminal illness. We knew we needed to be strong for them and give them hope. It was something we knew we had to feel in our own hearts before we could share with them.

Arriving at Anastasia and Daryl's a few days before Thanksgiving I could feel all my motherly instincts getting ready to take over. There was no food in the house for the big dinner, and it felt like a heavy, dark cloud hovered over their condo. Something didn't feel right. Anastasia was edgy and short with everyone, especially me. She had been that way the entire time during the long-distance planning of her wedding. I never understood at the time that it wasn't me she was upset with. I was still taking things so personally.

So when I suggested we go grocery shopping together, she came and whined about having to serve turkey. Why not fish? She was a vegetarian and wanted fish. Robert was scheduled to arrive the next day with his girlfriend and dog, and he would want turkey. I couldn't handle the conversation calmly. Who cared what we had for Thanksgiving dinner? Dad had a terminal illness. Neither of them had discussed it or asked about it yet. I had it in my mind that it was the only thing we should be talking about. I was edgy with Anastasia and responded as a mother talking to her small child. "We'll have BOTH!" I heard myself yell.

Looking back I wish I had given her a long, big hug and said, "Is everything okay? What's going on?" But that was then, and I was still wrapped in my own emotions and thinking about life as if it was all about me.

Robert made his grand entrance from Boston later than planned. All of us, including the well-cooked turkey, were waiting for him. They had gotten lost, but they were finally there. Robert had always had the aura around him that the minute he walked in a room his energy was felt. The attention was his, and he loved keeping it. One couldn't help liking him with his stories and passion for life, yet the impact of his enthusiasm was exhaustion for everyone listening.

Dinner was a variety of vegetarian dishes, salmon, and the regular Thanksgiving dinner of turkey, mashed potatoes, gravy, cranberries, and apple pie. I was worn out. Someone else was doing the dishes, as I had cooked everything.

I thought I knew best. I thought I was thinking clearly. I thought I needed to protect Anastasia and Robert. I thought being the helicopter was a good thing. I thought it was all about me. I thought I needed to make the numerous lists and check things off. I thought I needed to take care of things. I thought all these things gave me some control of my life. That was then.

The conference was amazing. There were about 250 patients and family members present. It was very organized, with a guest speaker opening the conference with a welcome statement. We were given choices of workshops that we could attend. There were different doctors that specialized in certain areas of both diseases, Aplastic Anemia and MDS. Bob really wanted to attend the lecture concerning iron overload.

Iron overload occurs when a patient has many blood transfusions. As a patient receives blood he gets not only the oxygen carrying red blood cells but also the iron that is present. Iron deficiency is not an issue with a MDS patient. When they receive the red blood cells during a transfusion they eventually get too much iron and this is referred to as iron overload.

At the time we attended the conference there was only one way to alleviate the extra iron from your system (called chelation therapy). Chelation therapy consisted of having a pump attached to the patient at night that helped flush the iron out through the kidneys. Bob was interested in a new drug, Exjade, which was on track to be approved by the FDA. It was going to be offered as another option for chelation therapy.

As we interacted with other patients and families there was a statement that was said over and over to Bob: "Oh, you are still double digits!" The patients compared their counts like a group at Weight Watchers might compare the number of pounds dropped during the previous week.

The numbers that were being compared included red blood cells (RBC), hemoglobin (Hg), hematocrit (Ht), white blood cells (WBC), and neutrophils. The only number we were aware of was Bob's hemoglobin. It was 11.2. A healthy person's range is 13.0-18.0. We had ONE number that represented the MDS. It was his hemoglobin and it was a double digit! There were ample opportunities to sit and talk with other patients and families.

Story after story was shared by those attending the conference about how many years they had survived MDS with multiple blood transfusions. Stories of how the disease had progressed to include the white blood cells and even the platelets. Stories of how the treatments changed their bodies. There were stories from family members about how the disease had impacted them and their relationship with their loved one.

The mood in the car on the long drive home to the Rocky Mountains was different. We were both feeling fortunate and blessed. Our lifestyle might be slower, but we were going to live and enjoy each day. MDS might be a terminal illness, but we were ready to live each day to the fullest. Bob turned to me and said, "I think I want to get a dog!"

Angels do find us in our hour of need.

Amy Huffman

4. Angel

We had a dog when the children were growing up. It was a family pet that survived being around an active family and eventually was taken over with arthritis. Oreo had started out as a ball of fur when Robert and Anastasia were small and ended up saying good bye to us when Bob and I were home alone as empty nesters. We never considered another dog with both of us working so many hours and knowing retirement was right around the corner.

We always came together with lists for all the decisions we have had to make as a couple. We looked at the lists and compared notes and opinions. Bob's desire to get a new dog was no exception. When questioned why to get a new dog, I was not surprised with the answer. My engineer husband, being practical and logical, stated that the new dog would give him a reason to walk and exercise. I agreed, but also knew in my heart that a new puppy would bring unconditional love, compassion, and lots of licks to the house.

We didn't just go out and buy a puppy. Oh no. Not us. The list included what we wanted in a dog. First was size. We both wanted one that could be on our laps. We wanted a small dog with doable pickups on the walks. We wanted personality plus. We wanted a dog that loved **being** loved and loved **giving** love. We decided on a Cavalier King Charles Spaniel.

Oh! What a dog! We went and looked at her and fell in love. She was tri-colored and a little darling. We had to wait several weeks before we could bring her home, so we decided to think of a perfect name. The choices included Latte, Precious, Sweetheart, Love, and many more. One day while we were out running an errand Bob yelled out, "Angel!" I said, "Where?" I had no idea what he was referring to. "Angel, for the dog's name," he said. I just smiled and said, "Perfect!"

Angel came into our lives and turned out to be just that, an angel. She and Bob bonded from the first day. I drove and Bob held her close to him on the hour and a half ride home. From the first day it was obvious who was going to be number ONE in Angel's life. The pattern began early with Bob and Angel taking a walk every morning. After the walk, Angel would collapse on the cement deck while Bob had his morning coffee and read the newspaper.

The walks in the beginning ranged from forty-five to seventy-five minutes long. Bob wore a heart monitor to make sure he wasn't overdoing it. He always felt out of breath, but watching his heart rate was the safest way to make sure he wasn't in trouble. Bob had the desire to push, but he never pushed too hard. He knew how important walking was in the big picture of staying strong.

Bob's first blood transfusion of two units of blood happened about two years after he was diagnosed. It was a major event for us. We knew that the MDS was progressing, as promised. There was no magical calendar to follow. No lists to check off. It was going to happen on its own schedule regardless of how much exercise Bob did, regardless of how healthily he ate, and regardless of how much we prayed it would not progress. Bob had researched about blood transfusions and discussed with the doctor about having the blood ordered to be irradiated, leukocytes reduced, and CMV negative.

This special order would help alleviate possible issues in the future if he ever had a bone marrow transplant. Ordering the blood with these special guidelines made it harder and longer to process. He was confident it was the right way to go. Every transfusion he received from that day on, except for two, was blood that was irradiated, leukocytes reduced and CMV negative.

Bob's determination to remain strong and active made me look at myself and make some decisions about my own physical strength. I had never been a gym kind of girl. I always put my lesson plans, papers, committees, kids, and husband above my own needs.

There never was any time left to attempt things just for me. That's what I told myself at that time in my life. Once I was retired I had very little to blame for my lack of exercise. So I made up my mind to join a gym. The results were much more than loss of weight or inches. I felt stronger and great doing something just for me.

There was something else that happened at the gym that I had not anticipated. There were many women that I interacted with. There was a bond that developed. As I shared Bob's diagnosis, I found compassionate, caring responses. One day a woman I had briefly spoken to the day before searched me out and handed me a small book. She said she had been impacted by Bob's MDS story and our spirit. She asked me to please accept the book and invited me to go for coffee whenever I felt like it. That was the beginning of a wonderful friendship. That kind, generous woman was named Ruth. Angels come in many forms.

We cannot direct the wind,
but we can adjust the sails.

Dolly Parton

5. Adjustments

Our days continued on as new patterns set in. Bob enjoyed the daily walks as much as Angel did. We purchased a new oversized couch for the family room. The couch was needed so Bob could stretch out and take his daily naps in comfort.

We continued to discuss life in general and what we wanted to do with the time we had left. We both had accepted that MDS was a death sentence and we were no different than anyone else except Bob had a piece of paper with an estimated range of time before he died. It wasn't as morbid as it sounds. We decided to look at it as a chance to do and see some things. As long as those things weren't high-exertion activities, like hiking, biking, or tennis, we were ready to go. We decided to travel to Hawaii.

We had never been to Hawaii, and it offered all the things we loved: water, warmth, flowers, and relaxation. We decided on the island of Kauai after one of the exercise girls offered her condo at a special rate. She warned me that there was a steep hill to the beach, but that the complex offered golf cart rides up and down to the beach. It sounded perfect.

Perfect was not the word for our experience. As we sat and watched the sunsets and smelled the tropical air, our conversations continued to be of our time together, our children, and our time we still had. We purchased a timeshare the second day on the island and vowed, if it was physically possible, to return every year. I loved the promise we made and the peacefulness that I felt sitting next to Bob with both of us relaxed and calm. I wanted to always remember that calmness whenever I closed my eyes and pictured the palm trees and water.

The trouble with a vacation is that once home reality hits you in the face. Our reality came with a phone call from Anastasia. She didn't know how to tell us, but she was leaving Daryl. We asked for details, thinking it was the result of an argument or disagreement. As we listened we realized she had made up her mind. Bob told her he was flying out to talk to both of them. It was decided I would stay home with our puppy, Angel.

Within three days Bob and I knew the marriage was over. Anastasia had known before the wedding that things were wrong. She just didn't know how to step away. She was embarrassed and sad. I recognized the strength and courage it took for her to make that decision. We tried to support her long distance. Our conversations were frequent with little conversation concerning her dad's disease. There didn't appear to be an emergency of any kind, just her dad feeling tired all the time. Her drama took priority.

During one of the visits with the doctor Bob asked about having a bone marrow transplant. Bob had done some research and realized it was the only hope to possibly have the disease disappear. The doctor said there were several locations that performed the transplants and that he could see about setting him up with a consult. Bob had researched several and requested the one located in Seattle (www.seattlecca.org). It had the best statistics for success with MDS transplants.

Within a few days, someone called from our insurance company and had made an appointment with a doctor for a consult. Our flights were confirmed. We would travel one day and return the next day. We were elated! Maybe this was the opportunity and answer to our prayers.

The meeting was well organized with all of Bob's medical records in place. The doctor had read everything and proceeded to outline on a whiteboard the dynamics of MDS. The bottom line was that Bob had not progressed far enough into the disease to be considered for a transplant. His quality of life was better now than it would be by having the transplant. The doctor suggested we return when the disease progressed and his symptoms were much worse. Among the statistics shared were that for Bob's age (he was then sixty-two) there was a 25 percent chance of surviving the transplant. He also recommended having siblings tested to see if there were any matches available.

We flew home with what should have been excitement that Bob wasn't bad enough to have a transplant, but instead the adjustment we had to make was that he would get worse. He would get to the point where a bone marrow transplant was his only option. How long did we have? Was it worth considering an option with only a 25 percent chance of survival? Bob's only living relative, a brother, was tested. He was a perfect match. He passed away before his cells were needed.

By the next spring, Bob was receiving two units of blood once a month. The new drug for iron overload, Exjade, had been approved, and he convinced the doctor to let him begin taking it. The purpose was to try and keep his ferritin level down. Ferritin measures the amount of iron in the body. Exjade was a very expensive drug, seventy thousand dollars a year, but if it worked it was worth it. First thing in the morning for the next five years, he would grind the large tablets up and add them to a liquid and drink it.

We adjusted to the pattern that evolved around Bob's blood transfusions. The day of the transfusion meant a full day at the infusion room. The process took between four and five hours. I would pack a lunch for us, bring a deck of cards or a good book, and we sat in one of the dozen chairs in the infusion room. We got to know the nurses well, and I would make homemade goodies for them. They were our extended family.

I didn't experience the same panic then that I had felt three years earlier during our first time in the oncologist's waiting room. I understood that each patient was unique, and we were doing well compared to many of the other patients. Going home after the infusion was like taking a deep breath. We knew we were good to go for another month. We had a new pattern, or cycle as we referred to it. There was good energy, and Bob was pretty stable during the few weeks after receiving blood. It became the window of time to go and DO. We would go to dinner with friends, walk with Angel, grocery shop together, and go to movies ... whatever Bob wanted.

By the end of the third week his counts would begin the drop. We always knew this by his level of energy. His naps were every day and there were fewer trips up and down the stairs. Angel's walks were shorter and sometimes I would have to do them during the last few days of the cycle.

In the fall of that year, my father passed away. It was the first time I had witnessed a person die. There were many family members present, and one of the nieces would later comment on how I had "lost it." Looking back I did lose it. I remember holding my dad's hand as he died and having Bob's hand on my shoulder. I just kept thinking the whole time, how was I ever going to handle Bob dying? My chest hurt as I cried out in pain.

I knew it was time for me to talk to someone. The next week I made an appointment with a therapist.

*No one remains quite what he was
when he recognizes himself.*

Thomas Mann

6. Finding Myself

It might be hard to believe that I had never been to a therapist before. It wasn't because I had no reason to go. Maybe it was due to the fact I was too busy making lists. Who knows? I was committed to sit across from someone who was a professional and receive advice.

I look back on that first visit now and think about what thoughts must have been going through Maria's head. Here sitting in front of her was a middle-aged woman with notes written out. Yup! Maybe I even had a list, I can't remember. I came to Maria and told her my husband had a terminal illness and I was looking for some strategies for dealing with his death. It sounded SO logical and direct. Poor Maria! She had her work cut out for her.

Our appointments were once a month and lasted for the next three years. It was my new beginning. It seemed Maria would always end a session with a question for which I had no answer. I would then go home and ponder the question. The pondering caused me to look inside myself and discover not only who I was, but where I had come from. It was amazing what I discovered.

I reflected on my personality and where it had evolved from. The amazing thing is once I understood the life events that forged my being; I was able to leave those events in the past. I was truly happy with my core and who I was. I was able to see the good in being the helicopter. It brought me joy to understand my generosity. I felt empowered in my ability to say no and gifted with my skills of organization and creativity. I realized that I really liked myself and that I had so much to share. It was such a wonderful feeling to have confidence, courage, and love in my heart.

My sessions also impacted Bob. He had encouraged me to go to see a therapist. I had invited him to come with me, but that was not going to happen. "You go," he would say. "I don't have any issues I need to deal with." I still smile when I think of that conversation. He would drive me to the appointment and wait in the car with a good book to read. We would always go to our favorite nearby restaurant after the appointment.

As I got in the car after a session and settled in, he would start with, "How was it?" followed by, "What did you talk about today?" I would share some of the details and he would add his comments of "That's good," or "I agree," or "That is really a great question." He really was happy for me as I was more and more at peace. I recognized my peaceful response to him, inquiring about the session, represented a growth in myself. I wanted him to be part of me finding myself. He was so much a part of me.

I would forever be grateful to Maria for helping me in discovering myself. As far as the strategies on how I was going to deal with being alone, I never received answers. We never discussed any. It was about going home and loving Bob today, loving life today, sharing myself with family and friends today, and knowing that I had the strength, courage, and wisdom to face anything that came my way.

*We must accept finite disappointment,
but never lose infinite hope.*

Martin Luther King Jr.

7. Hope and Disappointment

Looking back the next two years seemed like a roller coaster. The high of the ride were the times we had hope that maybe we had found something to slow down the disease. The lows were the times Bob felt so disappointed and physically miserable.

There had been a new drug approved for the treatment of MDS. It had shown some success in studies to slow down the disease. Vidaza was a strong drug that had side effects. Bob discussed it with his doctor and they decided to begin the regime. It meant getting injections five days in a row and then waiting three weeks. The injections were done in the infusion room, and the nurses would always be suited up with masks, gloves, and gowns. The gear was to protect them against the strong drug.

They started with a half dose to see how Bob would react. It didn't take long to realize that the drug was attacking both his red and white blood cells. He soon became neutropenic. Neutropenia is when white blood cell counts go too low and the risk for infection increases. Low white blood cell counts come with a phone call from the nurse warning to wash hands frequently, stay away from sick people, not to pick up after pets, and avoid crowds. It was something that we would become way too familiar with.

Bob just felt awful overall. He kept hoping that when they finished the six-month regime that things would improve. Before the six months were completed the doctor convinced Bob that they needed to cut back on the strength of the Vidaza, as it was affecting his system too severely. He completed the six months and stopped it. During the whole time of treatment, our old pattern was nonexistent.

There were many events that I did by myself. Angel and I bonded as I was her partner for walks. All grocery shopping, lawn mowing, snow clearing, or anything that entailed using energy or being out in public was on my plate. I kept up with classes at the gym, but found I needed to have my exercising completed by seven o'clock in the morning so I could be available for doctor appointments. I found a spinning class twice a week that started at six o'clock in the morning. I never dreamed there were as many people on the same early schedule as myself.

Bob lost hope as the time passed and it became apparent that the Vidaza had not slowed down the MDS. The blood transfusions were just under a month apart. The number of units of blood that he had received was slowly adding up to be near the one hundred mark. I privately discussed his depression with the physician assistant (PA) at the oncology office. She astutely had a conversation with Bob and asked how he was sleeping and if he felt he was depressed at all. He answered, "Yes, sometimes." She asked him, "Do you want to do anything about that?" It opened the door for Bob taking an antidepressant. That was a big step for a guy who thought he had control of things.

We scheduled another trip to Kauai and realized that he was going to need a blood transfusion while there. He found that the air travel impacted his red blood cells, as it used up the oxygen in his cells. Bob went to work advocating and arranging the details of getting blood work done on the island and also finding a location for the blood transfusions. The logistics of organizing the blood transfusion were tedious. Bob took it upon himself to organize, communicate, and make arrangements. He was disappointed that the blood he would receive was not going to be irradiated. In order to have what he wanted he would have to fly to another island. Bob let go of that demand. It was yet another time he let go of control.

As another year passed the space between the blood transfusions reduced to about two weeks. The cycle that we had when they were a month apart was very similar. The only difference was that we only had about seven days to get up and go. Bob would start to fade by day eight or nine. We stayed close to home, and the daily chores became all mine. Angel, being the angel she was, knew when Bob was not feeling well and would find her spot at the top of his chair burrowed down by his neck. She was his pillow firmly attached to him.

Bob decided to try the only other drug on the market that was explicitly produced and tested for MDS. That one was called Revlimid. It was his last hope. The studies and clinical trials had produced great results especially with MDS patients that had a chromosome 5 deletion.

Even though Bob did not have the chromosome 5 deletion (his was chromosome 9), he felt it was worth the chance of trying the regime. The statistics were not available for patients with a chromosome 9 deletion. After a meeting and discussion with his oncologist, they decided to give it a try. "Here we go again," I thought. Another six months of agony and not feeling good. It would be worth it if it worked, meaning that it would slow down the disease.

One of the things that I found strange and annoying was that Bob seemed to always be the one to be searching out the next step in his approach to the disease. The health-care system seemed to be content with just keeping him going with his regular blood transfusions with no talk of possibilities. Was it a story I made up in my head? It didn't matter as the Revlimid was started. Bob was just days away from his sixty-sixth birthday. He had survived beyond his three- to five-year window he had been given when diagnosed. He had lived seven years with MDS.

Six months later, we both felt the disappointment. He had given it a good try. The doctor reminded us that maybe the Revlimid had really helped him. Who could know? Without it maybe Bob would have been getting blood transfusions every week versus every two weeks?

The Revlimid attacked his bone marrow. Now his white blood counts were so low that he was neutropenic all of the time. We were always afraid of Bob getting an infection. We knew it could kill him. We carried hand soap with us wherever we went. We limited our company to those who were healthy with no fevers or runny noses. Bob stopped attending holiday dinners with family. That was the time in our life to reflect and celebrate the support of friends and family. We would never have made it that far without them.

*Let us be grateful to people who make us happy,
they are the charming gardeners who make
our souls blossom.*

Marcel Proust

8. Gratitude

Gratitude is a simple word. Feeling gratitude is humbling. Expressing gratitude is essential in the process of feeling it. My gratitude toward the people in our lives during the MDS years is indescribable. I know we would never have made it through our journey without the support and love of those around us.

We picked our house online before ever seeing it in person. It was located on a cul-de-sac with a beautiful tree in the middle of the road. There were only nine houses on the cul-de-sac, and there was evidence of all different ages being represented on the street. We could see the mountains and a lake from our back patio.

Some of the first neighbors we met were Jackie and Jack. They introduced themselves to us, and we knew we would get along with them. Jackie was a sweet woman with a kind and compassionate disposition. Jack was a retired engineer and hit it off with Bob immediately. They eventually invited us to belong to a dinner group that they participated in. This dinner group was made up of couples that had been friends for many years. The dinners were at their homes and sometimes at a restaurant with dessert at someone's house. Regardless of where the dinner was held, the company was genuine and enjoyable.

Jackie and I developed a very special friendship. We both had an interest in scrapbooking and recording memories. I had done nothing with thirty-five years of family pictures. They were in boxes labeled *PHOTOS*. They were not sorted by event, child, or even dates. What a project! Kimberley, my sister-in-law, was a consultant for a scrapbooking company and had given me a basic scrapbook starter kit for my birthday.

Bob had been diagnosed by the time I received my starter kit. I began the mission to record all of the memories I had with Bob, the kids, and myself: the old ones and all the new memories we made from that day on. Anyone that enjoys scrapbooking knows the job that was ahead of me. Just getting thirty plus years of memories organized and recorded is monumental. I had all the activities we did day-to-day to put into albums and record. We didn't know how long we had to be together. I wanted Bob to be able to sit and look at the past memories with me and to be part of what I referred to as our retirement adventures. Scrapbooking became my therapy in many ways.

Jackie and I made a pact to scrapbook once a week. We picked Mondays as our special day. We would break for lunch and continue on until dark. We loved the time together. She was a wonderful listener but shared her stories, too. If I was in a panic or feeling fearful about Bob she would calm me or let me vent. She heard about my therapy sessions and would support me as I sorted through everything. It was amazing how fast those days went by.

We decided to open the scrapbooking up once a month to the women in the dinner group and others who would enjoy the opportunity. I bought expandable tables and set up half the basement as our work area. Kimberley became our consultant and we had a great time socializing and scrapbooking. Even my mother, who was in her eighties, joined the group and started organizing her years of photos.

As Bob's disease progressed our scheduled Mondays were always up in the air. We knew the time was on the calendar but understood if anything happened it would be pushed to another date. Jackie and the girls understood and remained flexible. We stopped having lunch upstairs because Bob couldn't be around crowds. The girls would bring their bagged lunches, and we would take a break and have a picnic lunch downstairs. This support system was amazing. This was a group of genuine, kind, and supportive women. I would close my eyes many times and say, "Thank you."

Jackie and Jack were a special team for us. After our scrapbooking on Mondays, the four of us would go out for dinner. We girls loved it as we didn't have to cook, but more than that it was the opportunity to bond as couples. We invited them to come to Hawaii with us and share paradise. It was the best trip we had taken to Hawaii. We took about 800 pictures between us, and the guys got so tired of us saying, "Wait … we HAVE to have this picture!" We shared sangrias, kalbi, salmon burgers, and our favorite tacos. The memories and special time together was part of the bond that made them our forever friends.

Another forever friend was Ruth. Since the day at the gym when she had given me the book and invited me to coffee, I knew she was special. Ruth was a wise and good soul. Her compassion and love of life was contagious. She respected that I did not have the freedom to pick up and go like she did. It made our time together even more special. We had many serious discussions about books, movies, beliefs, politics, and my favorite … religion. She was the friend that would be there at the drop of a hat if I needed her. I knew I would always be there for her, too.

My mother supported us in her own unique way. She existed only for her children, and she was happy when they were happy. I didn't share all the details of Bob's disease with her. She would take on all the details as if she were living them, and sometimes I think she would suffer more than those struggling. She loved being kept in the loop of all the news and would put Bob's transfusion dates on her calendar.

We would sometimes leave Angel with her on the transfusion days. Mom was Angel's second mommy. When it came to Mom, I just wanted to be part of making her happy. I helped her in the garden, with setting up family dinners, and with decorating and cleaning her house. I was there for whatever she needed help with. We had a wonderful bond, and I felt it was a gift sharing special time with her.

My large family did the best they could to be supportive of Bob and me. I always felt that the baggage from our childhood was a wall that some of my siblings just couldn't climb over. I was second oldest of the tribe, and admittedly I was left in charge many times when we were young. Bossy could have been, and probably was, my second name. There was always competition between the siblings. There was some jealously. After being away from family for thirty-some years, being in the pot was a new experience for me.

I had much gratitude for all the support that was so steadfast and generously given to us. I had gratitude for the love and kindness that surrounded us. I had no idea the role and importance this network of friends and family were to become in our lives.

Once you make a decision,
the universe conspires to make it happen.

Ralph Waldo Emerson

9. A Decision to Make

On Labor Day weekend, when Bob was just a few months from his sixty-seventh birthday, we found ourselves flying back up to the beautiful Pacific Northwest. On Tuesday we arrived in Seattle at the same clinic we had visited some years before. That time Bob was at a different place with both the disease and his mental state. He was ready to actually see if he was a good candidate for a transplant. He knew he was ready, but he didn't know if they would think of him as a possible candidate.

A doctor we had never met before had Bob's file in front of him. I was surprised to see how thick it was. There had been several more bone marrow biopsies completed after that first one eight years before. He had all the records about frequency and amount of blood transfusions. It was all there. The doctor's conversation sounded encouraging about a transplant.

The one statement that rang like a loud bell for both of us was the fact that Bob could die sooner from an infection than from MDS. His low white blood cell counts were dangerously low and made him very susceptible to infections. His body would have trouble fighting any infections. The doctor was amazed that Bob had not needed to visit any emergency rooms in the last two years in regard to him being neutropenic. Most neutropenic patients have visits to the ER with infections and fevers.

He told Bob that his age could be a factor and that there were many tests that had to be completed and passed before a transplant would be official. Bob talked statistics with the doctor and discovered that the chance of a patient his age surviving a transplant had increased from 25 percent to 35 percent. There was more data available because there had been more transplants since our last visit.

The one fact that the doctor was very excited about was that Bob had a blood-related donor who was a perfect match. Bob just stared at the doctor. "No, my brother died four years ago." The doctor replied, "I'm so sorry for your loss." No one had updated the records. That would make a big difference as a donor would have to be found, which could take weeks or months. The doctor left the room and said he would start a search on the worldwide bone marrow donor site to see if any donors popped up as possible matches. In the meantime we were to meet with a representative from the financial department.

The financial representative was full of information for us. There were some questions she could not answer and referred us to the guru of finances, Q, as he was known. Q was out of the office, but we could call him anytime. The stress point for Bob was the ambiguous answer to the question, would Medicare pay for it? We were hearing the answer, "Well, some patients just put up the money upfront, and then Medicare reimburses." This was not the answer Bob wanted to hear. It was clear he needed a yes or no. We did not have the three- to four-hundred thousand dollars to put upfront. Bob was a numbers kind of guy. Finance was always black and white.

The doctor returned with the news that there were thirteen possible candidates in the computer. These possible matches would need to be tested to see if they matched Bob. "Should we start the search?" asked the doctor. Bob just stared at him. Would Medicare pay for it? We did not have that answer, and Bob couldn't say yes to the go-ahead for the search without confirmation on the finances. Bob told the doctor he would call when he had made up his mind.

We toured the facilities, which included meeting with a head nurse who explained the team concept. Bob would be assigned a team of doctors and one head nurse. We toured the nearby teaching hospital, and we saw where patients from out of town lived. A volunteer drove us back to the airport, and before we knew it we were back home.

In a twenty-four hour period of time, our lives were turned upside down. We returned home with many questions and an overload of information. We spent time with Jackie and Jack going over all the data and material. They had many comments and questions that helped Bob process the overload of information. It was so good to have friends to help sort through everything. The truth was Bob had a decision to make.

If opportunity doesn't knock, build a door.

Milton Berle

10. Fight!

I never dreamed that Bob's fight for life would start with a mammoth fight with the insurance company. I have since learned that we were not alone with the challenges that arose when dealing with big insurance companies. That was to be one of Bob's biggest fights of his life.

After our visit and consult, Bob went right to work on gathering information concerning the coverage of a transplant. We were part of a large HMO that managed his Medicare coverage. So the first place he went was to the HMO to get some questions answered. That was easier said than done. Every phone call ended up with him being transferred or referred to another person. Keeping track of phone conversations, people's names and phone numbers, and information received was something he expected to do.

We finally received a call from a transplant coordinator within the HMO that said, "No, we won't cover it and neither does Medicare." Bob was napping that day when the phone call came in, and I remember saying something like, " ... And that is it?" She apologized, and I couldn't stop talking. I just started venting. I don't remember my exact words, but I do remember the tone and emotion that I spoke with. I asked why, and she replied that Medicare doesn't cover transplants for MDS. They covered other diseases, but not MDS.

"WHAT! Are you kidding?" I was livid. So I summarized my interpretation of the news for the person on the other end of the phone, "You are saying that Medicare patients with MDS won't be covered because ... because they are too old and they don't want to spend the money to keep them alive, because they don't have that long to live?" I continued sharing the emotional stress that Bob had gone through just to make the decision to try for a bone marrow transplant. I told the woman on the other end of the phone that I knew it wasn't HER decision, but still, what devastating news. I assured her Bob would want to discuss it with her when he woke up.

Bob's conversation with the insurance representative was a repeat of mine. The difference was that Bob was not full of emotional statements. His words were clear, concise, and determined. He informed the representative that he would be appealing the decision.

Bob worked for weeks to prepare the appeal. It included copies of his medical record, a letter from his current oncologist encouraging him to have the transplant, results of studies, and last but not least a personal letter. As I watched him prepare this appeal I realized the emotional toll it was taking on Bob. The day after day work of compiling all of the information and sharing his emotions of life and death in black and white was exhausting and very difficult. The reality of the importance of the timing of having a bone marrow transplant became so evident. It was now or never. The window of opportunity was closing quickly.

Bob asked me to read the appeal packet before he mailed it. It was a thick document written from the heart of a sick man with a mind and soul of an engineer. I read the personal cover letter first. The last paragraph brought tightness to my throat and tears to my eyes. I had to reread it.

In summary, I have no hope of altering my steadily deteriorating bone marrow disease and suffering further loss of Quality of Life if I continue to rely only on supportive care. I am willing to participate in an appropriate clinical trial and I believe that offering me a chance at survival through an Allogeneic Hematopietic Stem Cell Transplant is a humane and compassionate treatment plan. Consequently, I am appealing to you to approve coverage for an Allogeneic Hematopietic Stem Cell Transplant. Time is of the essence to approve coverage for my HSCT before I deteriorate much further.

Never had I seen such a clear description of feelings from someone who was dying and clinging to hope. A copy was made of the appeal, and it was sent on. It was early November.

We heard back on December 10. There was a time restriction on the HMO for how long they had to respond to the appeal. They responded on the outer limit of that time restraint. It was a single-page letter stating after reviewing the appeal the decision held. Bob looked up at me and said, "Now it goes to Maximus." Maximus represented Medicare and would review the appeal. As always, Bob had his plan in his head long before that letter arrived. He knew he would appeal to Medicare on the HMO's decision. It meant another four to six weeks for an answer.

The holidays were upon us again and Bob was even more exhausted. I pulled out the decorations and arranged them to present a holiday mood. Each year I had done less and less with decorations. It had gotten harder and harder to accomplish the heavy hauling by myself. The mood was heavy as we realized Bob's options were getting fewer and fewer.

The week after Christmas, Bob discussed that he thought we should get our will in order and go do as much as we could in the next year. He was quiet, but determined to have things be in place and in good order for me when he was gone. We had paid off the house a few years before. It was a silly thing to do in the economy at the time, but a necessary thing in his mind.

He insisted I take over all the bills and finances. It wasn't something that I had refused in the past, rather it was something he never wanted to let go of. He gave up having to drive everywhere and would just get in the passenger side of the car on the days he didn't feel like driving. All of these signs served as a clear image of what was going on inside Bob.

I remember the day we decided to sit and work on the will. We were in the office and filling in our wishes as each question came up. We were doing both of ours at the same time. The details of what we wrote down were really not important. I will never forget the burning in my eyes as I listened to him so logically go through everything. He was so matter-of-fact about his decisions, and I knew he was feeling at peace knowing that this was getting completed. His desire was to make sure things were lined up and in order to make my life easier when he was gone. My eyes burned from tears of sadness and the deep love that I had for him.

One's destination is never a place,
but rather a new way of looking at things.

Henry Miller

Big Sur and the Oranges of Hieronymus Bosch

11. A New Mindset

Bob adopted a new mindset to enjoy life while he could. So during the holidays we decided to make reservations for Hawaii in April. It gave us something to look forward to, and we both realized it might be our last trip there together. The hassle of getting blood transfusions while visiting paradise didn't faze us anymore. It had become part of our life, and we accepted all the efforts of executing the details. Bob voiced a desire to get away from the winter climate. I made reservations for the month of February on the beach near San Diego at a pet-friendly condo. Angel would come with us.

Bob went to work on making the arrangements and connections for blood transfusions while in the San Diego area. We had visited California before and found the blood transfusions very difficult to arrange. There were more hoops to jump through in California then there were in Hawaii. He somehow lucked out, speaking to a nurse coordinator in San Diego who seemed to be very familiar with what needed to be done. She organized the details and kept in close communication. She proved to be our angel in San Diego.

We decided to drive to California. It was hard on Bob to fly, and we would have more freedom to accommodate Angel. We have always loved our road trips. We packed our special items to make our month comfortable, and off we went to share peaceful and relaxing time together. The condo turned out to be perfect. It was comfortable, on the ocean, and very pet friendly. It also had a gym and a hot tub. There were almost as many pets as people in the development. The first week we were at the condo the letter arrived from Maximus stating that Bob's appeal was denied. The transplant would not be paid for.

My mother came to visit for a week or so. It was awesome having her relax with us. She enjoyed a glass of wine while watching the sunsets, took walks with us, and just enjoyed sharing special time. When we were due for our first transfusion she stayed with Angel at the condo while we went to the hospital. It was great.

My friend Ruth was able to come and stay with us, too. She had an event in the area and extended her stay to include special time with us. I believe this trip expanded our friendship to include Bob. We did things together and enjoyed sharing with each other. One of my brothers, Charles, visited the area, and we were able to see him and socialize with his friends. Anastasia lived in California and was able to spend long weekends with us. She brought her dog and Angel loved the extra company.

I made a special birthday dinner for Anastasia. I included all her favorite foods and surprised her with pearls from our last trip to Kauai. We had not had many opportunities in the past years to celebrate birthdays together. It felt like we were entertaining from our home away from home. I found myself at peace and loved each moment I shared with Bob.

Bob spent some of his time reading and surfing on the internet. He was searching for any news of studies or new ideas that might get him the transplant. He ran into a new study that had just started about a month earlier. It was looking for 250 MDS patients, sixty-five years old or older, who would be willing to participate in a study to see how long they survived after a bone marrow transplant. Yes, it was being run by Medicare.

I didn't believe my ears when Bob read it to me. I made him repeat it several times. "Are you kidding?" was all I could respond with. Where was the HMO? Where was Medicare? Why hadn't someone let him know about that study? How could it be that a study had just started seeking participants exactly fitting Bob's condition?

The study was not for a new drug, but for the survival period of a transplant patient. It was amazing! It was a true miracle.

Bob used his time making calls. He started with the HMO. No one knew anything about the study. Even though he had the study's name and ID number, no one knew anything. He tried calling the university where the data was to be collected. He talked to the woman in charge of collecting the data. At least the study was **real**. She informed Bob that the transplants could be done anywhere in the country as long as the facility agreed to complete the paperwork involved. There was a limit of 250 participants. Bob asked her how to get signed up, and she was not sure.

It was like we were in *The Twilight Zone*. Here we were so close, but no one knew details of how a person was to jump onboard. Bob broke down and called the cancer clinic we had visited for the consult. He talked to Q, the financial guru. "Yes, we are aware of it. We have two patients right now participating in the study." Bob took a deep breath before asking the next question. "Is Medicare really paying for it?" The answer was simply, "That is our understanding." The only issue Bob had was who he needed to talk to in order to become part of the study.

Don't be afraid to see what you see.

Ronald Reagan

12. Turning Point

It was the last week of our month-long beach vacation. We had arrived with a mindset that Bob's terminal illness of MDS was closing in on his precious time on earth. Our goal was to keep making wonderful, peaceful memories. We accomplished that goal on that trip. By the end we had news of the new study, and there was a ray of hope again that maybe, just maybe, Bob would have a chance at a transplant.

The next morning we were due at the hospital for his last blood transfusion before we hit the road to go home. We were gradually starting to pack things up for the long trip. Bob had mentioned a sore back a few days earlier and had been applying heat to it. What was I thinking not looking at it? While getting dressed for the hospital I asked him how his back was feeling. He commented, "Still sore." I walked over to see if I could see anything and about had a heart attack.

There on his back was a cyst the size of an egg that was inflamed and red. I knew it was infected. Infection was the scariest word in my vocabulary. I tried not to overreact with a scream or gasp. "Honey, that must be so sore!" and "How long have you had the bump?" were all I could get out of my mouth. We were on a time restraint to arrive at the hospital on time for his blood transfusion. I collected things for our four- to six-hour adventure in the infusion room, knowing I was going to have a nurse take a look at his back. Bob was calm and said, "Just don't make a big deal about it."

After Bob got settled in and hooked up to his blood, I started looking around at the crowded room. We had met the nurse coordinator at our last transfusion. I had made our appreciation for her professionalism and extreme compassion known. She was a hugger, so I added a big hug to our verbal thanks . I had asked for her business card so I could write a letter to her supervisor, commending her.

I looked around the nurses' station to see if our angel nurse, as I referred to her, was there. My eyes scanned the room and found her over at a computer. I apologized for my interruption and told her about the cyst and asked if she could help us out. She examined the spot on his back and said, "We generally call this an angry cyst, but I would call this one a really *pissed* cyst." It **was** bad. Even I could see it was getting bigger and redder. She left us alone, and when she came back she told us that Bob would have to go to the ER after his blood transfusion. The cyst would have to be examined, probably lanced, and treated.

We sat in the infusion room thinking about poor Angel back at the condo. There was no one I could call to let her out or feed her dinner. We had assumed we would be back in time. With an ER visit we knew it would be hours before we would be able to attend to her. It was yet another time in the MDS journey that I took a deep breath and asked myself, "What is the worst that could happen?" My answer to myself that time was a mess to clean up and a hungry Angel. It was going to be okay.

I don't think I sat in the infusion room thinking, "What is the worst that could happen with Bob's infection?" I didn't want to go there. I had experienced tightness in my chest only one time before when I thought about the worst that could happen. That was a few years prior when he had an x-ray and it showed he had phenomena. I sat there getting flushed and light-headed and could feel the tightness in my chest. It had turned out okay, but I decided then not to make up stories ahead of time about the future. It took too much energy.

I also discovered that when we were around nurses and hospital staff I let my guard down. By that I mean I let those professionals take care of all the health issues. It had taken years for me to allow myself to do that. I discovered finally that if I emotionally let go of his care when professionals were near, it allowed me to breathe and relax and take a mini break. Sometimes I would even leave him and take a walk, browse the hospital gift shop, or talk to someone on the phone. Little lessons learned.

As we signed in at the ER, I immediately thought of germs. It had become my life. I made Bob put a mask on, and we tried to sit where there were the fewest people. We were in for a long wait. After a few hours I stepped outside and called my good friend, Jackie. She was a retired nurse and always the good listener. I told her the facts about the cyst. It was an old sebaceous cyst Bob had for years that must have gotten infected. I know she heard the fear in my voice. She was amazing as she thought out what the next days would look like. She advised me to find out explicitly how to dress the wound, what medications should and could be applied, and even told me to get some supplies given to me before leaving the ER. She reassured me that I could do anything that needed to be done. It was exactly what I needed. It was a calm and commonsense approach.

About three hours later we were escorted to a small cot with a curtain around us. I knew enough that Bob couldn't have food or drink until he was seen. He was getting thirsty and hungry. When the doctor finally arrived and looked at the cyst on his back, we were both ready for him to fix it. He was impressed with how big it was and laid out his sterile kit on the bed and asked Bob if he would mind if he took photos.

He said he was a teaching doctor and it was a classic example of a very infected sebaceous cyst. Bob didn't care what he did. There was no nurse helping the doctor, so I asked if he minded if I watched. I couldn't believe I was standing next to him watching the procedure. I was amazed at myself. I remembered Jackie saying I could do *anything* that needed to be done. I knew it was time for me to step up and be able to handle seeing blood, procedures, and all the other medical obstacles. I even put gloves on and handed the doctor some more gauze.

We were sent home to the condo with instructions that Bob should be seen the next day by a doctor to change the bandage. They had taken a culture to discover what kind of infection was present. He was put on some antibiotics. Bob and my conversations were all about infection and how soon could we get home to our own health care provider. We were given the name and location of a clinic near our condo to go to the next day. Bob's plan was to check out of the condo, go to the appointment, and then travel north to spend the night at Anastasia's. We would then hit the road for home.

The next day at the clinic the change of dressing showed a lot of drainage. The wick was taken out and a new one inserted. I was not going to be changing the dressing as long as there was a wick involved. It was a painful procedure to replace it. The new doctor asked me how the wound looked compared to the day before at the ER. I drew a circle with my finger where the cyst had been. Not much difference in size. He took a marker out and marked the outline of the redness and said this would help the doctor who saw him the next day.

We left the clinic with the same instructions to see a doctor the next day. We started the drive north to Anastasia's. The phone rang and it was a nurse from the ER from the day before. She had another prescription to add to what Bob was already on. They did not have the final results from the culture but did not want to take a chance, so they were going to cover all the bases. We checked on our iPad to see where the pharmacy nearest to Anastasia was located. We drove straight to it and waited the hour and a half to have it filled.

Bob was beat by the time we arrived at Anastasia's place. The last time she had visited us at the condo all was well and her dad had taken a walk on the beach with her and the dogs. She was in shock at how whipped and out of it he was. We called Robert to update him on the happenings and he yelled, "Get him on a flight home, now!"

Why hadn't I thought of that? Bob had just kept talking about driving home and how we could do it. It was late in the evening, and I knew it was going to take until the next morning to convince Bob to considering flying.

The next morning Anastasia came with us to the local ER. We were the first ones in the lobby, but it still took an hour or so to get in. The doctor changed the dressing and discussed Bob's MDS history and the saga of the cyst with him. I asked what the doctor thought about Bob driving back across the Rocky Mountains. Bob interrupted and said, "I can do it!"

The doctor didn't give an opinion, and said he wanted to talk to someone from the ER back in San Diego. We waited a long time and went back and forth debating about Bob making the trip in the car. Anastasia finally asked her dad if he would do what the doctor recommended. "Yes," Bob replied. The doctor returned and said they still did not know what kind of infection Bob had. The way he handled the question of driving was very diplomatic. "If it were my father, I would put him on a plane and fly him home immediately." Well, there you had it. The decision of flying was made.

By early afternoon a flight had been made for Bob to fly out and arrive home by evening. Robert would pick him up at the airport and spend the night with him and deliver him to Bob's primary care physician first thing in the morning. I took a deep breath and let out a sigh of relief. My plan then went into action of getting Angel and me home.

The car was still packed from leaving the condo the day before. I called Judy, my sister, in Las Vegas and asked if she would be home that night. I told her the plan to spend the night with her and leave at the crack of dawn to try and make it home the following day. I had never driven the trip by myself. Bob and I had made the trip many times but always shared the driving. One of my fears was hitting snow going through the Rocky Mountains.

As I backed out of Anastasia's driveway she leaned into the window and commented that she knew how I felt when I sent her off to college, with the car all packed up and a long road trip ahead of her. "Be careful, Mom, and be aware of people around you when you stop at gas stations. Don't make eye contact with anyone!" It was great advice that brought a smile to my face.

Angel and I made a great team on our long trip home. I played and sang along with my *Mama Mia!* CD most of the way and realized if it hadn't been for ABBA I might have fallen asleep at the wheel. Whenever the wheels went over onto the bumps on the right side of the road, Angel would lift her head and ears and look at me as if to say, "Mom, what are you doing? Stay on the road!" I knew she really was my angel.

The whole episode of Bob's infected cyst, ER visits, emergency flight home, and my solo drive home changed me. It was a self-realization that I could handle whatever came my way. I reflected while driving home that we came very close to what the doctor had said to Bob at the consult, "You will die from an infection before you die from MDS." I felt a renewed fear grip my heart. I also felt a new courage inside me. I just knew that I was strong enough to face whatever the future held.

Little did I know what that was going to be.

Impossible situations can become possible miracles.
Robert H. Schuller

13. Making Lists

I think the episode of the infection changed Bob, too. Within days of getting home Bob called and left a message for the doctor that he had seen at the cancer center in Seattle. The message was, "I am ready to be part of the study. Please add my name to the list of candidates and inform me of what I have to do." Within a day or so the response came telling him to be sure and let the HMO know he was going to join the clinical study. The doctor would have someone contact Bob from the Donor Department to let him know what the next step would be.

Most of the phone calls to the HMO concerning the transplant proved to be both frustrating and exhausting for Bob. In the past every time he would get off the phone from talking and/or yelling with the HMO, he would almost be shaking and the color was out of his face. At this point of time I knew Bob was frustrated and angry. He had dealt with appeals, runarounds, and unreturned calls. At one time he had complained to the State Insurance Board to investigate the fact that the HMO would not address questions about travel and lodging in connection to a transplant.

The gentleman dealing with the complaint, Mr. J, told Bob that he had discussed the issue with a member of the HMO and that they would move forward with Bob's request. When Bob called the woman at the HMO office she denied having the conversation with the gentleman from the State Insurance Board. At that point Bob just replied, "Really? You never have spoken with Mr. J, from the State Insurance Board? Thank you for your time. You will be hearing from the State Insurance Board." He had let go of yelling or trying to talk to a supervisor and released it to another higher authority. I felt he was saving his energy for the bigger battle.

The phone call to the HMO to tell them he was going to join the study was one of the most determined conversations I had ever heard Bob have with the HMO. He simply called the number listed in his Evidence of Coverage Package (EOC). According to the EOC, he had to call and let them know he was going to be part of a clinical study.

So the conversation was one-way. Bob gave his name and ID number and told them according to the instructions in his EOC he was informing them that as of today he was joining the clinical trial and gave them the number that identified the study. The next thing I heard him say was, "That is not my problem, I am following the procedure set forth in the EOC." He hung up and my hand slid down his shoulder and I rubbed his back. With relief in his eyes and face he looked at me and said, "It has started."

Within a few days Bob received a phone call from a friendly, informative woman from the clinic in Seattle. She represented the donor search. She answered every question that Bob could think of and told him that they would take the top six possible matches and begin the more involved testing to see if any were matches. "Why only six if there are thirteen possible matches?" asked Bob. It was explained that it was very costly to do the intensive testing on the candidates and they only did them in groups. It made sense to start with the strongest possibilities. She informed Bob that it would take three to six weeks for testing. If there was a match, we might only have two weeks to arrive at the center for the beginning of the process.

Our emotions ranged from fear to excitement. I think the thing we felt most in our hearts was hope. Hope that there really was that **one** donor out of a possible million candidates listed in the worldwide donor website. One out of a million was not very good odds. We both held hope for the possibility.

Needless to say, we went into action. We immediately started our lists. We had lists for packing, list for doing, and lists for issues that needed to be communicated with both the HMO and the clinic. Bob suggested we start putting anything we wanted to take on the dining room table. That way we could judge if it would fit in the car. We felt we would need to take our car for transportation while at the clinic. I was in charge of the list for fact finding for places to live. I couldn't commit or make a reservation, because we didn't know if we would even be going, so it was just fact finding. I discovered that rent was going to be about three thousand dollars a month and it included parking for the car.

Bob's list was detailed and extremely long. It was handwritten with bullets out in front of each item. There were dozens of items. He had several eight by eleven inch yellow pieces of paper laid out on the counter. Both of our lists were results from reading a booklet that was sent to us titled, *Getting Ready for a Bone Marrow Transplant.* The window of time to plan to be away from home and at the facility was four to five months. Four to five **months**! That was a long time to shut down our house and lives. Who would have guessed there were so many details and things to do? Part of Bob's list included:

- Stop Paper
- Find Lawn Service
- Forward Mail (Once we knew the address.)
- Get Current Medications Filled
- Take All Medical History for Bob
- Stop Internet Service
- Buy Cell Phones (We only had one at the time.)
- Stop Comcast Service
- Set Timers on Sprinklers
- Buy an iPod Speaker System (Music for our room.)
- Get letter from HMO stating they denied payment of travel/lodging expenses (They had refused to put in writing and we needed it to file an appeal.)

- Get letter from HMO stating they would pay the 20 percent of costs after Medicare payments
- Power of Attorney
- Organize Folders for Receipts, Medical Information, and Bills ...
  Bring Birth Certificate (How somber that was. It was in case Bob did not survive the transplant.)

My list had travel arrangements and domestic issues:

- Find a place for Angel
- Cancel flights/lodging to Hawaii in April
- Thermometer (Foods had to be cooked to certain temperature.)
- Open a Blog on CaringBridge (www.caringbridge.org) to use for Communication between Family and Friends
- Favorite Recipes
- Favorite Protein Bars and Snacks
- Baggies of Seasonings needed for Recipes
- Addresses of Family and Friends
- Birthday and Anniversary Cards needed for four to five months
- Scrapbooking Supplies
- Exercise Mats and Bands
- Baby Gifts for three new babies due during time gone

We would check off things done on the lists, and before we knew it we were adding more. It was very intense.

After about four weeks we heard from the donor center. None of the six candidates they tested had matched. Our spirits were shattered. Bob asked what was next. He was told that there were only four candidates left to test. She encouraged him not to get discouraged. There were always new entries into the donor bank. She said one of the donors wouldn't be available for a week to test and it took ten days to run the blood work. So the earliest we would hear back from her would be three weeks.

We slowed down for a week on the lists after that phone call. Then we realized that if a miracle occurred and there really was a donor that matched Bob, we better get moving on checking off items. That was a time I refer to as being driven. Both of us were intense about everyday activities and rarely took time to smile or acknowledge each other.

It was at that point I added something right in the middle of Bob's list. With a bullet in front of it I wrote, "Tell your wife you love her." Later that day when I was out running an errand I received a text message from Bob that read, "I love you--check." It brought the biggest smile to my face, especially the word check. We would use the word check many times in the months ahead to simply tell each other how much we loved one another.

The next phone call came late in April. They had found a match. Not **perfect**, but a nine out of ten match. The donor was a twenty-seven-year-old male from Europe. That was all they could tell us. The Miracle had happened. They wanted us in Seattle at the cancer clinic for our first appointment on May 17.

Don't be dismayed at good-byes.
A farewell is necessary before you can meet again.
And meeting again, after moments or lifetime,
is certain for those who are friends.

Richard Bach
Illusions: The Adventures of a Reluctant Messiah

14. Saying Good-bye

We knew it would be fast-moving when we heard about the donor. Suddenly it was real. One of our biggest stresses was Angel. What to do for four to five months with Angel? I looked online and found an agency that would place her in a loving home. Anastasia and Robert were not available to watch her. Anastasia had the limit of dogs on her lease already. Robert was traveling and running a business and did not have quality time for his own dog. All of my siblings had their own life issues that just didn't fit into a long-term commitment of adopting Angel.

At the time my mother was dog sitting during the day for my sister's two mini dogs. They were brothers and one was two years old and the other eight months. They would be dropped in the morning and picked up after work. There were gates up to confine the pups to the linoleum. My mother had said she would watch Angel, but she also expressed stress from the commitment of the two she already had. I knew I could not add another dog into the mix. Once the call came from the cancer clinic giving us about two weeks to arrive, I sat with my Mom and had an honest, emotional conversation.

She had watched Angel in the past whenever we went to Hawaii. As a last resort, I knew we could always put Angel with the family I had found online. After the heartfelt conversation, my mother insisted Angel stay with her. She would tell my sister it was time for her to take over watching her dogs. Bob and I committed to an amount to pay her every month even though my mother protested. Bob and I spent the afternoon before we left with my mother and Angel. My dear mother would be our angel forever and she would become Angel's number-one mommy.

Saying good-bye to all our friends and family was not easy. At the time, Bob and I knew the statistics for surviving a transplant. A person his age with MDS had a 35 percent chance of surviving. We carried this number in our heads and hearts. As we said our good-byes, everyone knew there was a chance that Bob might not come home. It made the hugs and last dinners even more memorable and emotional.

I held one more scrapbook day with the girls, and we cried and shared the special time to the fullest. Bob and I took Victoria and Cayman, our niece and nephew, out for hamburgers and fries. They were aware that Uncle Bob was sick. They could not come over if they had a cold or a runny nose. They knew that their uncle took naps a lot and sometimes when they came over to the house they had to be really quiet. We explained to them that Uncle Bob was going to go to a special place that was going to try and make him better. We would be gone for a long time, but we would text them and talk. We loved the smiles and hugs we got every time we saw them.

The exercise group sent me off from the last spinning class with cards, hugs, and gifts. Ruth invited Bob and me over for a special dinner. We spent as much time as possible with our good friends Jackie and Jack. We had an extra copy of the booklet about preparing for a transplant and gave it to them so they could follow the timeline of our happenings. I could see the stress and concern in the eyes of everyone as we said our good-byes. I tried my best to reassure them that all was going to be just fine. I asked all of them to keep us in their hearts and prayers.

Those thoughts and prayers were going to prove to be our lifeline.

A wise man adapts himself to circumstances,
as water shapes itself to the vessel that contains it.

Chinese Proverb

15. 450 Square Feet

We left home on a beautiful day in early May. It happened to be the day of my good friend Ruth's seventieth surprise birthday party. Her daughter had been organizing it, and all of us were keeping secrets for a month. It was going to be quite the party. I gave her extra hugs in the days before our departure. I missed celebrating with everyone, especially Ruth.

The drive to the Pacific Northwest took us through three mountain ranges. The scenery was some of the most beautiful I had ever seen. It took us two and a half days to make the trip, with me driving all but three hours of it. Bob needed a blood transfusion as soon as we could get one. Once we left our home, we looked forward and found ourselves not worried or thinking about all the lists and issues we had focused on for the previous two or three months.

I had made reservations to stay at a facility run by the cancer center. It was only two years old, and our first impression was how clean and bright it was. There were rooms of different sizes labeled as patient, caregiver, and family rooms. We had reservations for the caregiver room and within a week we moved into a family room on the fourth floor. It had a hide-a-bed couch, queen-size bed and a twin-size bed.

There were no walls separating the space, and it was designed for handicap accessibility so the bathroom had no tub, just a shower with a seat. The room did have a microwave, sink, and two small dorm-size refrigerators. We thought if Robert or Anastasia visited we would have room for them. The room was less than 450 square feet. Our home we left was 3700 square feet, so the apartment felt quite small. It got smaller as the months progressed.

All real cooking was done in a community kitchen. It really was a very well-thought-out facility. There were eight individual cooking areas with pots and pans and utensils. Against the wall were restaurant-size refrigerators and freezers to store food. Everything had to be labeled with our name and room number. We were assigned locked lockers where we could store our canned goods or staples.

The rules of the kitchen were simple. Everything had to be washed after use and run through one of the sterilizing machines. Gloves had to be worn while putting the dishes away. The sponge had to be sterilized after each use. The rules were in place to protect all of the immune-suppressed patients staying at the facility. My average time for preparing any meal and cleaning up was about one to two hours.

The kitchen was just one community room located on the second floor. There was a resource center that had two computers and a printer. The entire floor had windows that wrapped around the outer walls. The view included the downtown skyline and the Space Needle. Tables were set up that followed the outer edge of the windows that held half-finished 500- and 1000-piece puzzles waiting for the next person to come and sit for a while.

The media room had about a dozen movie seats with a big screen. Movies were available at the main desk to sign out. The exercise room had a large area with mats, weights, exercise balls, mirrors, and a bar across the mirrors. Off from the main area was a smaller room that held two NuStep training bikes. I had been diagnosed six years earlier with very little cartilage in my kneecaps. I found the best medicine for my knees was riding a bike. I had never used a NuStep before, but knew we were going to become friends.

Also on the second floor was a beautiful children's room full of toys, puzzles, and games. The entire room was brightly carpeted. There were balloons, and the whole atmosphere was bright and cheery. Outside the children's room on a long bench was a full life-size marble black lab. I found myself sitting next to the statue and petting it. The children's room was used by patient's children, grandchildren, or visitors. Only once did I see a child use it that was a patient. Most of the children with cancer were staying at a different facility closer to Seattle Children's Hospital.

The first floor was where the office for check-in was located. The staff was amazing when it came to helping out with questions or concerns. That was where the vacuum cleaner, movies, DVDs, and almost anything needed could be found. The eighty units had mailboxes located on the first floor, along with a conference room for staff meetings. The room I was going to get to know the best during our stay was the laundry room. Located on the first floor, the room held eight washers and dryers stacked nicely. They were free and were in use most of every hour of every day.

The seventh floor was the roof of the building. It had lounge chairs and tables with umbrellas for patients and families to go and be in a quiet, open place. The roof was planted with wild flowers and sedum and felt like a garden in the middle of a city. It was so eco-friendly. The minute the elevator door opened to the open air of the roof, I always felt myself take a deep breath. It was as if I was entering a calming aura and relaxing place. These special surroundings would prove to be my safety net in the months to come.

It was amazing how a place could feel like home so quickly. Even though it was less than 450 square feet, that apartment would be our home away from home. It would prove to be a protective and safe haven for us as we faced the unknown.

Courage and perseverance have a magical talisman,
before which difficulties disappear and obstacles
vanish into air.

John Quincy Adams

16. Tests and Specialist

Bob and I settled in and were anxious to begin the meetings with the doctors. He was ready to get going on the transplant. Our first meeting was with the two lead doctors and Nurse J, who would be part of Bob's team. One was a visiting doctor from Texas and the other was on staff. We found out that the staff doctor was from the same town on the East Coast as we were. We exchanged stories about the cold and snow. It was a pleasant visit with a physical and going over Bob's history with MDS. One of the first discussions circled around the drug he was on, Exjade. He had been on it for five years to help flush the extra iron out of his system. All those blood transfusions had played havoc with his ferritin level. The doctor was concerned about his creatinine level so the first official order we received was to stop taking the Exjade.

Blood draws would be done regularly and they would be watching his counts. Bob was concerned about getting the blood work done and blood ordered for his needed transfusion. He was dragging and knew he needed one. He also knew that back home it could take three days to get all of the work done and schedule the transfusion. Nurse J picked up the phone and made a call. Within five minutes he was scheduled for a blood transfusion on the fifth floor of the same building.

This organization and efficiency was amazing and comforting. We knew we were in good hands. As the meeting progressed we never felt rushed or on the clock. It was about getting to know Bob and Bob getting to know them. The last question the doctor asked Bob was, "How do you feel about being here for a transplant?" I sat there and anticipated his answer being, "A little nervous" or "Apprehensive." Instead Bob smiled and said, "I am very excited about being here. I have the hope that this will cure me!" The doctor smiled.

Our days were filled with schedules set out by the clinic. We were assigned a team, Red, which meant the Red Team of doctors and nurses would follow us until discharge. The doctors would rotate monthly, but our head nurse, Nurse J, would be with us forever. Her name and number was entered into my contact list on my phone. She was my go-to person for concerns, questions, and advice. Another angel had entered into my life.

At the main desk on the transplant floor, there was a file or mailbox especially for Bob. We would check this red file every day to collect revisions of our schedule or information we needed or a document that needed to be signed. I loved the organization and the feel of having a team that knew what they were doing, communicated to us, and had the compassion to listen to even the smallest concern or question. It felt like we had arms around us from the first day.

The days filled up quickly with what were referred to as pre-transplant tests. We knew they were all needed to make sure Bob was strong enough and to be sure all his organs would survive the transplant regime. Before we arrived we hadn't realized that he had to pass all these tests before he would get the okay to go forward. We just assumed it was a go--not so. Just because there was a donor waiting for the okay to collect his cells didn't mean it was going to happen. They had a tentative date of June 7 on the calendar for the transplant. We learned early on that anything on the schedule is only a plan. In reality, life and appointments are taken minute-to-minute. Flexibility and adaptability were lessons I would learn quickly.

Some of the tests were difficult for Bob. The pulmonary test was one of them. His breathing had been impacted by the MDS and the level of oxygen in his blood was always compromised. As with everything Bob attempted, he did his best. I watched as he blew through the tubing and turned red and then white as a ghost. He had chest x-rays, a MUGA test, blood work galore, a prostate evaluation, two bone marrow biopsies, and of course a visit to the dentist.

Bob's history with his teeth was not a happy story. His mouth was not his best feature. He had issues way back when he was in the Coast Guard. Maybe it was genetics, it really didn't matter. There were issues he had been dealing with for years. The goal of the dental visit was to make sure he wouldn't encounter any infection issues within the first year of the transplant.

That first year is a delicate time and having teeth worked on is not recommended, so they try to anticipate any problems and take care of them before the transplant. The dentist was a kind, gentle woman. As I watched her examine Bob's mouth, I saw her brow wrinkle when she looked at his records then back to his mouth. I knew she had found something. "Bob, I want to send you to the university dental school to have them check this one tooth. It shows a small spot, and I want to make sure it is not serious." Bob listened intently and agreed. Neither of us was too worried, as he had seen his regular dentist just before we left and felt confident that there would be no major issues.

Scheduling the dental appointment took a few days. It was our first visit to the University of Washington Medical Center. It was about a ten-minute ride from the clinic. The hospital was enormous with maps available of each floor to help you navigate through the maze. We checked in and were escorted to a cubical where a dentist examined his mouth with the tooth in question being the main concern.

The assistant had placed a pair of black sunglasses on Bob to protect his eyes. He wore a Hawaiian shirt that day, and I commented he looked like Jack Nicholson. I was trying to keep it light. The dentist and assistant laughed, but Bob was not amused. The news was not good. The tooth in question had decay already near the gum. It would have to be pulled. I couldn't see Bob's face, but I knew by the tightening in his arms and shoulders that he was upset.

More bad news followed. The dentist explained that there was another tooth that needed to come out because it had a cavity. That tooth was part of an existing bridge. They would have to cut the bridge, and then remove the tooth. The plan was to file the bridge where the cut was made and Bob could have any dental work done he wanted a year after his transplant. There was no choice. We left with two big gaps in Bob's very sore mouth.

Bob accepted the teeth pulling with the attitude that it was only teeth. I was proud of his ability to pop back from bad news and go forward being positive. We met with the Red Team a few days after the teeth were pulled, and they questioned how he was doing. Bob repeated that it was all part of the big picture. With the tentative date of the transplant quickly approaching, Bob focused his questions about details of the date. It was then that the team hit us with some disappointing news.

Bob's creatinine level was still elevated. The team was concerned about his kidney function. To be sure that all would be well after the transplant, they decided to send Bob to a kidney specialist. The tests also showed a speck of blood in his urine. He would also have to see a urologist. The appointments with the kidney specialist and urologist would take another week or two to schedule and get the results back.

The donor would have to be notified that there was at least a week delay on the transplant day. We wondered if there was a way to go ahead and collect the cells and store them until after the appointments That just wasn't going to happen. Once the stem cells were collected from the donor, it became a time crunch to get them transported to us. We discovered there was a narrow window of time from the collection of the cells to having the cells infused. So our anticipated June 7 date was no longer.

We had to wait until the next team meeting to hear the results and reports. There was more disappointment. When the cancer center had contacted the donor center to delay the harvesting of the stem cells, it was communicated that the donor wasn't available the following week. We would have to move the transplant date to June 30. Bob was so disappointed. He was anxious to get things started. The next few weeks were continued lessons in practicing flexibility, adaptability, and patience.

*There are some things you learn best in calm,
and some in storm.*

Willa Cather
The Song of the Lark

17. The Calm Before the Storm

I made regular journal entries on our CaringBridge blog. It was a great way of communicating and sharing feelings and facts of our journey with friends and family. I found writing the entries was therapy for me. It allowed me the opportunity to organize my thoughts and emotions. Looking back, I realize I filtered the fear or anxiety I felt. The journal helped me keep positive and hopeful. It was not only appreciated by those reading it, but I found the guestbook comments encouraged and impacted us. It brought support, love, and prayers from all who were keeping track of us.

Monday, June 6
Bob and I keep looking at each other and referring to this time as the "Calm before the Storm". It is quiet, but we know what is coming.

We have met several patients that have had transplants and they refer to their progress as "Day 11", or Day 20…" One couple, Wally and Helen, are on Day 21. We see them regularly at the blood draw and have caught up with their story. Helen and I have been emailing and the other night she made the comment that we should be enjoying every minute that we can be "out". Her advice is as long as Bob feels well enough to go out to eat, or sightsee or whatever, DO IT! Since Day 0 they haven't left their room except to visit the Clinic. Wally hasn't felt like eating and is weak and sleeping most of the time. With that wisdom and advice we have taken to the streets of this beautiful city.

Wednesday, June 15

We got a call this morning telling us that a message had been received from the Donor Center and due to "donor availability" the Transplant has been put off, again, for another week. Our disappointment cannot be described. Anastasia will fly home this Sunday and come back later.

Today the Hickman line WAS put in. Bob did well. It took about 3.5 hours to complete whole process.

So, the new schedule is:
Sunday, June 26-Chemo
Monday, June 27-Chemo
Tuesday, June 28-Chemo
Thursday, June 30-Total Body Radiation and then TRANSPLANT!

All I can say is I am learning to put everything on the calendar in pencil.
Let's all pray that this is really the date. We are getting tired of waiting.

The weeks of extended waiting were difficult for Bob. He was **so** ready to just do it. It had been many months of preparing both mentally and physically for the actual transplant. We both at times would let our imagination go wild and think about the donor. Maybe he was not sure he wanted to do the procedure and just got cold feet. Maybe he had a wedding to attend and just wasn't available to process his cells.

My imagination was a little more flamboyant. I imagined the handsome twenty-seven-year-old European, with wavy black hair pulled back in a ponytail, taking a planned week-long motorcycle ride with his friends. I found myself thinking to him, "Be safe and stay healthy." We finally let it go and just accepted that the schedule day for the transplant was June 30.

We decided to enjoy what time we had. Bob still was receiving blood transfusions about every twelve days. Other than the time in the infusion room for blood transfusions, there was little time we had to be at the cancer center. We were just waiting for the process to begin. One day Bob asked if I would like to take a ride. He had not driven since we began the trip to the cancer center in May.

I was the driver, and he was the navigator. He said the day trip would be a surprise and away we went. Bob directed me about forty-five minutes north into beautiful country. There were mountains to the east, north, and west of us. The countryside was green with rolling hills. We both enjoyed viewing the water that was everywhere.

Our destination was a casino located in the middle of nowhere. We were not big gamblers, but Bob loved the buffets. Whenever we visited a casino back home I loved the poker machines, and my biggest splurge was maybe twenty dollars. When I pulled up in front of the casino, I knew Bob had brought us here to make me happy. I knew in my heart we should not be there. With Bob's counts so low, we had no business being around crowds and eating from a buffet.

The team at the clinic would have heart attacks if they knew. I smiled as we arrived and said how nice it was that he was trying to make me happy, but that I didn't think we should go in. Bob reassured me it would be okay. I decided a fast lunch with no gambling would be our plan. An hour later we were back in the car. I made up my mind that our casino stop would never make it on a one of my entries on CaringBridge.

I started to turn south to return home, meaning our apartment back near the cancer center. Bob announced he had one more stop. Instead of going south, we continued heading north. We only went about ten miles and exited westbound. Fifteen minutes later we crossed a bridge and arrived at a beautiful island. We drove around the entire island, and Bob asked me to pull into a real estate office.

We met with a young, friendly agent named Keri. Bob inquired about the weather, cost of living, prices of homes, and lifestyle on the island. We left the office with a map and some current listings and drove around looking at available homes. We loved looking at houses wherever we were visiting. On the way back to our apartment, Bob asked me if I could move to the area. I had no answer. He couldn't be serious thinking of a move with everything ahead of him.

We acted like tourists for the next few weeks. Bob only had energy to do one outing a day. We visited the popular places in the area, ate at different restaurants, and took pictures of everything and every place we visited. I was writing all the details on CaringBridge. DJ, a friend from back East, commented on the website after seeing all of our pictures. "If I didn't know the story of why you are in Seattle, I would swear you were there on vacation."

The art of simplicity is a puzzle of complexity.

Douglas Horton

18. Logistics

The logistics building up to the actual transplant were mind boggling. It was like putting the last pieces of a giant puzzle in place. On the donor's end, the cells were collected. That process consisted of the donor receiving a drug ahead of time that boosted his production of stem cells. The drug, Neupogen, can cause some ache and pain in the muscles and bones.

The actual collection of cells was like a donation of blood, but it took about five hours. The blood went through a special machine and the cells needed were separated and saved. The blood then was returned back to the donor through another tube. It was very time-consuming and depending on the amount of cells harvested a second day could have been required.

On Bob's end it meant three days of chemotherapy, a day off, and then full-body radiation on the day the cells were infused. Once the transplant was definite, a Hickman line was surgically placed inside Bob's chest and connected directly to the entrance to his heart.

The Hickman was developed by Dr. Robert Hickman, a pediatric nephrologist at Seattle Children's Hospital. The purpose of this invention was to make blood draws and infusions painless and effortless. The placement of the Hickman required surgery, and I wasn't allowed in the room to watch. Up to that point I had never left Bob's side during a procedure. Every test, every blood infusion, every event found me close to him.

Anastasia was visiting us during the week right before the transplant. I remember the nurse telling us to go get coffee and he would come out and get us when the procedure was done. I walked down the hall with Anastasia with tears on my cheeks. She asked me what was wrong. I had to think why I was crying. It was that helicopter in me. I had been with him 24-7 since arriving at the cancer center six weeks earlier. It was time to release the care of Bob to the nurses and doctors, and let it be.

Once Bob came out of surgery, he was quite perky. I think he was **so** happy to finally be on track for the transplant. The nurse was the first male nurse we had met since arriving. He was a yogic, gentle, deep-breathing kind of guy. He instructed Bob on the mechanics and care of the Hickman. The clear dressing over the place of entrance was to be changed once a week. The two tubing lines that hung out from his chest had little caps on the end of them. They would need to be changed daily, and the tubing would have to be flushed with a solution daily.

The Hickman would have to be completely covered for showers. The disposable shield used for showers was called an AquaGuard. The nurse also explained that it was very important that Bob wore a cord necklace they supplied. At the end of the cord was a clamp. The clamp hooked onto a small cloth bag that the ends of the tubes were placed in. It was to serve as the emergency clamp to shut tubing down if bleeding occurred. There were lots of instructions and information. I knew Nurse J and the team would help us out with any questions.

Chemotherapy was to begin the day after the Hickman line was placed inside Bob. He had never received chemo before. The two drugs he had received previously, Vidaza and Revlimid, were not considered chemo. They were considered immune-suppressive drugs. Bob knew the chemo would begin to kill his marrow so the donor's cells could move in and set up house. On the morning of the first chemo procedure, we were met by a friendly experienced nurse. Nurse M listened to Bob's story and shared hers. Her husband had a bone marrow transplant two years before.

Hearing her story, along with her professionalism, helped make the first chemo infusion less stressful. She was amazed that

Bob had not had any chemo in the past. I pulled the camera out and asked if she minded if I recorded this first chemo experience. Nurse M had a mask, gown, and gloves on, but I felt her smile as she posed for the picture with Bob. That special nurse with her kindness and gentleness would follow us through the journey and become yet another friend and angel.

Bob survived the first session of chemo without any side effects. By the end of the third day, he was tired and worn out. He slept most of the time and just felt miserable. We expected that reaction. The fourth day was a rest day, and even though Bob physically felt terrible, he was in good spirits. He knew he was on the road to the transplant. It was really going to happen.

Tuesday, June 28
Bob started feeling the effects of chemo yesterday afternoon. He has diarrhea, a severe headache, tired, achy body, loss of appetite and generally feels worn out and sick. He has been in bed all day. He just finished a milkshake and is still in bed, resting. We keep reminding each other what the chemo is doing in combination with the drugs. It is getting his body ready for the new cells on Thursday.

Anastasia and Robert arrive tomorrow for the BIG DAY.
I will update when he has the new cells!!

Happiness is speechless.

George William Curtis

19. Happy Birthday

Transplant Day arrived and started with Bob spilling his morning hot coffee down his leg. His leg immediately turned red with pain. Anastasia and I applied cold compresses over and over, hoping to help with the pain. We hoped that the incident would not affect his full-body radiation that he was due to have that morning.

The radiation treatment took a short time. Within a few hours Bob was feeling really crummy. He had the chills all over and could not get warm. The team had him go to the infusion room, and they scheduled an IV of hydration. I remember arriving that day at the check-in desk on the infusion floor and having the receptionist behind the counter check him in.

The process was answering the questions, "What is your name?" and "Your date of birth?" After Bob answered those questions, a wristband was put on him. Bob was then handed the little beeper. It was similar to the gadget given at a restaurant while waiting for a table. It would buzz and flash red lights when it was Bob's turn to go back into the infusion room.

After putting the wristband on Bob, the receptionist disappeared and returned with several warm blankets. She started wrapping Bob from top to bottom with blankets. I remember thinking, what a compassionate thing to do. He looked like a mummy and didn't care when I asked if I could take a picture. By now he was used to me documenting everything with a picture. I already had filled one scrapbook since May when we arrived. That picture was one of the last before he received his new cells.

Anastasia stayed very close to us during the week building up to the transplant. Robert arrived that day. He said there was no way he would miss the biggest day in his dad's life. All of us were in Bob's infusion room waiting for the magic time of seven o'clock in the evening. That was the time we were to go to the hospital and check-in. The cells were to arrive on a plane that evening and be transported to the hospital. We could have had the procedure done in the infusion room of the cancer clinic, but they only stayed open until six. It was normal for donor cells coming from Europe to arrive late in the evening, so it was common for an overnight stay in the hospital.

Bob was weak and cold when we arrived at the hospital. Anastasia pushed her dad to his room in a wheelchair while I parked the car. I only knew about one parking area and used the maps to find my way. Robert arrived, and we all gathered together and talked with the nurse about the logistics of receiving the cells.

The nurse assigned to Bob was a calm and experienced woman. She answered all our questions. The day a transplant patient receives the new cells is referred to as Day 0. That day began the count for posttransplant tests and activities. The goal was to be discharged by Day 100. The first day, Day 0, marks a new birthday for the patient. It was June 30 and his cells would be infused into the next morning, or July 1. We all decided that his new birthday would be July 1. The nurse stuck her head in the room about ten o'clock and said the cells had landed. They were in the city and being processed. We all felt the excitement. It was really going to happen.

The nurse brought the bag of stem cells in at about 10:40 PM. She handed them to Bob and asked, "Would you like to take a few moments and bond with your new cells?" He held the bag in his hands and just stared at them. Everyone was speechless as they watched Bob hold the bag of cells. There wasn't a dry eye in the room.

This was it. The bag was hooked up, and they began their journey into Bob with a steady drip, drip, drip. We all just stared in amazement. The nurse checked in regularly, and about halfway through the process she arrived with all the nurses on the floor and a big poster all signed by the nurses that read, "HAPPY BIRTHDAY." There were many pictures that night of Bob, Robert, Anastasia, myself, and the nurses. It **was** quite a birthday celebration.

Don't forget to be kind to strangers.
For some who have done this have entertained
angels without realizing it.

Hebrews 13:2

20. The First Days

Morning came with reality facing all of us. Some of the excitement had been replaced with exhaustion. Robert had to hit the road to return home. Anastasia had one more day before she had to return to her job and life. We all had anticipated Bob would be released from the hospital by noon. That was what we were told the normal timeline was. I knew from our journey so far that normal did not exist. I learned early on about flexibility pairing with patience to accomplish one day at a time.

Bob was not discharged that day. His blood test showed an extreme elevation in is uric acid count. We had no understanding of what that meant or why it was happening. The hospital team wanted to keep a watch on him. They ordered countless tests on him and watched him like a hawk.

The next morning a young, sweet girl came to the door of Bob's room and knocked. She asked if he would be interested in a quilt. She was shy and spoke softly. I got up and walked over to her and greeted her. She held up a few quilts and asked if he had a favorite color, and he picked one. We both thanked her. Bob unwrapped the plastic wrapping around the quilt. The quilt was absolutely beautiful. It fit perfectly on Bob's lap and was just the right weight to keep him warm and comfortable.

It wasn't until the next morning when I was folding it that I saw a small note sewn on the corner of it. It read, "This quilt was lovingly made by the volunteers of the Stone Soup Quilting Ministry, a ministry of North Seattle Friends Church (Quaker). It is yours to keep. May it bless you and warm your spirit as it comforts and warms your body. God's love. Peace."

I walked over to the window and looked out with tears in my eyes. I had spent the night on a cot in Bob's room. Anastasia was due to take a shuttle to the airport that morning. She stopped to say hello before leaving. In the short hours it had been since she had seen her dad, he had changed.

He was retaining fluids and swollen. His face, hands, neck, and legs were all a new size. She was quite concerned and asked, "What is the issue? Why is Dad so swollen?" We explained that the level of uric acid was extremely high, and also he had been receiving hydration. The combination was causing him to retain fluids. We knew we were in good hands.

One of the doctors stopped by and talked to Bob, Anastasia, and me. He told us that Bob had received a phenomenal donation of cells. He had received four times the amount a patient usually receives. FOUR times! The cells were having a party within Bob's marrow and made the uric acid go crazy. He told us they would give Bob a one-time injection to bring the level down and get it under control.

They would monitor him very carefully. I was glad that Anastasia heard the explanation, as it helped her understand. As she was leaving she picked up the quilt and commented how nice it was. She pointed out that the colors of the quilt were just like her dad's marrow. The overall pink color she thought represented the whole marrow. The red color was like the red blood cells, the cream color was like the white blood cells, and the green she thought of as platelets. I would never look at that quilt again without thinking about Bob's new marrow.

I stayed one more night at the hospital, sleeping on the cot. I woke up at five in the morning and made up my mind that I needed to take better care of myself. I needed a shower and clean clothes. That was one of those times I had to look at the big picture and let go of trying to be and do everything. Bob had tried to convince me from the first night to go home. Home had become a relative thing. The apartment certainly did feel like home compared to the hospital.

I gathered my bag of belongings and made my way down the elevator to the floor that would allow me to walk over the enclosed bridge to the parking structure. I had parked there the evening of June 30. It was July 3 already. We were already past Day 0, Day 1, and were on Day 2! Only ninety-eight to go! Those were my thoughts as the elevator opened and I was greeted by a large sign barring the entrance to the pedestrian bridge. "This bridge is closed due to the holiday. It will reopen on July 5."

Great. Now what would I do? I hardly knew my way around when the bridge was open. I felt a little panic set in as I wondered if the car were locked in the garage. I wondered if I could even get into the garage. I felt the tears coming. I was exhausted and used up. On any other day I might have taken a deep breath and pondered my choices. That day there was not much patience or reason left in me.

I heard a man's voice as I was shuffling through my folder for the maps of the hospital. I turned to see a tall, well-dressed gentleman standing and reading the sign. "I have never seen this bridge closed," he commented. I replied, "I think it is due to the holiday." I knew he was as surprised to see me as I was him. It was five thirty in the morning on a holiday weekend. No coffee or gift shops were open. It was just the two of us.

He said he knew a way to get over to the garage and said it would take some walking. I followed him to the stairwell, and we started down. For just a split second I knew I shouldn't be following a strange man down a stairwell, regardless of how reasonable he seemed. I let go of the instant of fear as he asked why I was in the hospital. I told him Bob had received his transplant a few days before.

By then we were walking along a narrow tunnel located underground. He talked softly and gently the whole way about how fortunate Bob was and how he wished us only the best. As I looked down the tunnel I saw a familiar elevator. It would take me to the garage and my car. I sighed as we came closer to the elevator and told the stranger that I knew where I was. I turned to say thank you and he was gone. I turned a 360 degree circle to see where he could have disappeared. There was a flight of stairs to my right. Wouldn't I have seen him walk up them? I knew it was not by chance that I had been guided to this elevator. I got in and pushed the button and looked up and said out loud, "I get it! Thank you for the angel."

Have patience.
All things are difficult before they become easy.

Saadi

21. Fourth of July

The next few days were a blur. Bob did not feel well. He had gained about twenty pounds in less than a week. He didn't look or feel like himself. The added fluids affected his blood pressure and other organs. I watched as the staff at the hospital collected and analyzed data. I got into the routine of leaving around seven thirty in the evening and driving back to the apartment. I would do laundry, email, banking, and shower. I was back by six thirty the next morning so I could check-in with the night nurse to see how the night had gone.

During the five days at the hospital, I observed the efficiency, professionalism, and compassion that the entire staff showed to Bob. It impacted me. I found myself letting down my guard as I did in the past whenever he got a transfusion. I let the nurses be on and I found myself being off. I filled my time reading or surfing the internet, searching for houses for sale on our favorite island.

There was one issue that I found I had anxiety over. Bob was on a tremendous amount of medication. The amounts and prescriptions were changing day to day, and there were restrictions of foods, times, and interactions with other drugs. The nurses would come in so many times within a twenty-four-hour period and deliver his meds in a small cup.

They would stop in, what felt randomly, and ask if he would like a milkshake. I learned one of the medications had a window of time in which he could have calcium products. The nurses would identify the drug by name as they handed it to him to take. I sat and felt overwhelmed as the shifts of nurses changed and the medications continued to be delivered. I began to panic, wondering how I would ever be able to keep them all straight with their restrictions.

One day I asked the nurse, "How do caregivers keep it all straight?" She responded with, "It's easy once you get into it." I thought about her answer and knew easy wasn't the answer I wanted. That night, back at the apartment, I was thinking and worrying about the drugs and my huge responsibility.

Out of nowhere a comforting thought came to me. I compared my learning about the drugs being similar to my students learning math in my math classes. Mathematics represented high anxiety and fear to some of them. They entered the class with the fear of not being able to learn or be successful. I reflected how I encouraged them to take it step-by-step.

I knew as a teacher that once I found the method that made sense to that student, they would have success. Once they had success, they would build their confidence to where the cycle of learning would blossom. I knew it worked. I had seen it in so many students. The pride, the confidence, the joy of accomplishing something they didn't think they could. I knew I was the scared, nervous student this time. I felt the fear of not being able to do it. So I decided to ask the nurse for a printout of all Bob's medication. The next day I had a new level of energy as I walked into Bob's hospital room. I had a plan.

The nurse smiled when I shared my comparison of me to a scared math student. I asked the nurse if I could meet with a pharmacist. She said she would pass on my request. She informed me that the pharmacist always met with the patient and caregiver with the medication list before being discharged. I didn't want to wait until then. I needed to be able to look at the printout while Bob was receiving the medications. I needed to be able to ask questions and make notes. The pharmacist came in later that day with four typed pages of medications. There were columns across the top of the page that were labeled: Name, Purpose, Schedule and Comments,

7-8am, 9am, 11am-1pm, 2-4pm, 5-7pm, 8-9pm, and 10-11pm. Below each column were all the drugs that Bob was taking.

Name	Purpose	Schedule and Comments	7-8am	9am	11am-1pm	2-4pm	5-7pm	8-9pm	10-11pm
Cyclosporine (Gengraf) Do not remove capsules from foil packet until ready to take.	Prevents GVHD	Take **225 mg** every 12 hours. Do not drink grapefruit juice. **On the morning of the cyclosporine lab check, take your morning dose after blood draw.** Lab draws: **Tues & Thurs**		X two 100mg caps + one 25 mg cap				X two 100mg caps + one 25 mg cap	
Sirolimus (Rapamune)	Prevents GVHD	Take **1mg daily** **Take at least 4 hours after cyclosporine.** Do not drink grapefruit juice. **On mornings of Sirolimus lab check, take your morning dose AFTER bleed draw.** Lab draws: **Tues & Friday**			1 pm 1 mg				
Mycophenolate (Cellcept), MMF	Prevents GVHD	Take **1000 mg** every 12 hours. Best taken on an empty stomach. May take with some food if nauseated. **Do not take within 2 hours of dairy products, calcium containing foods, ORAL calcium or ORAL magnesium supplements.**	X 7 am Two 500 mg tabs					X 7 am Two 500 mg tabs	
Dapsone	Prevents Pneumocystis pneumonia	Take 50 mg twice daily		X Two 25 mg tabs				X Two 25 mg tabs	

All I saw were four pages of strangely named drugs with special instructions and times that had to be followed. It was yet another time in my life that I learned how strong, courageous, and capable I was. I would become efficient, knowledgeable, and confident as I once again went into the helicopter-mode of hovering.

Bob finally stabilized to the point that the hospital staff decided he could be released. It was the Fourth of July, and he was scheduled to see his Red Team at the clinic the next day. I drove him home to the apartment, and I felt nervous and edgy. I knew that I had left the security of the nurses and doctors checking on him and being responsible for him. It was now up to me. Bob went straight to bed and slept for hours. I checked on him, took his temperature, and gave him his medication at the right times.

I left Bob that night to go to the roof of our building to watch the fireworks. There was going to be quite a display on the lake by the clinic. Being on the roof gave a wonderful view of the celebration. I looked around at all the people around me. All were patients and their families staying at the housing facility. All were dealing with cancer in some stage or another. The patients were generally the ones sitting with blankets wrapped around them.

I stood close to the railing by myself, exhausted. I couldn't help but wonder where would we be next Fourth of July. Would we be celebrating Bob's one-year mark? Would I be by myself? Those thoughts still crept into my mind, especially when I was tired or Bob was not doing well. That night was one of those times. I closed my eyes and took a deep breath. That night was about the beauty of the fireworks and the celebration that Bob had new cells growing in his body. Next Fourth of July was a long ways away.

Too often we underestimate the power of a touch,
a smile, a kind word, a listening ear,
an honest compliment,
or the smallest act of caring,
all of which have the
potential to turn a life around.

Leo Buscaglia
Love: What Life Is All About

22. Waiting for Engraftment

When Bob was asked what he remembered about the time from when he received his new cells until he engrafted he would just say, "I don't remember much other than it was Hell!"

Engraftment is when the counts for the white blood cells (WBC) start moving up. It represents the donor's cells taking over. There was no magical timeline for this to occur. From other patients we met, we knew it could take up to three weeks. We just prayed that engraftment would take place. I kept our friends and family updated on our blog. Sometimes I felt I was giving too many details, and other times I left things unsaid, knowing the fear or exhaustion I felt could be read between the lines.

Friday, July 8, Day
I thought I would state the good things so far about where Bob is in this journey:
No nausea or throwing up, still able to eat, is able to take all his pills with water without gagging, doesn't have the chills as often, takes care of all his showering and personal needs on his own, believes in his future of being well and is pushing hard to eat and exercise.

The bad things he is experiencing at this point:
Exhaustion--he is always tired and drained. He has constant diarrhea. His taste buds are lost and we hope they find their way home. Things that used to taste yummy, have no taste and some things are very spicy

to him. Oh, did I mention tired and weak and just overall not feeling good?

Bob has been pushing and pushing to walk and build muscle. He tries to do more today than yesterday. On Day 0, at the hospital, he walked 142 steps. Today he walked 2372 steps! Tonight he wanted to get his pajamas on and I asked if he could do one more lap on our floor. He groaned and gave me the evil eye, but got up and did it.

The nutritionist wants us to aim for 67 grams of protein a day to help his muscle growth. When I give him a suggestion for choices for food I always include the protein value of each and give him time to decide. He always chooses the one with the most protein. What a trouper. I am recording his entire fluid and food intake daily. It helps when the doctors, nurses or nutritionist ask about his fluid or food intake to have it written down. My brain is so numb I don't think I am remembering much these days.

At the team meeting today I asked a few questions about what to expect (that's where I learned about the white cells being the first to show engraftment) and asked how they felt Bob was doing? The doctor just looked at Bob and said, "Remarkable". That says it all.

Tuesday, July 12, Day 11
There isn't a lot to tell you today about us other than we are moving through each day very slowly with one step in front of the other. Bob had his worse day, so far, last Sunday. He slept most of the day and barely got through the daily needs of eating and showering.

He also received his very first unit of platelets on Sunday.

Monday was a good day with eating lots of protein and walking again. Today is slow with a long nap this afternoon. He ended up getting another unit of platelets today and was crossed and typed today for 2 units of blood tomorrow.

Bob's biggest issue, other than exhaustion, is diarrhea. The one drug he is on is known for having this side effect. Poor Bob. So yesterday he was prescribed, "Boston Butt Cream". I thought it was a joke...why "Boston"? When I went to pick it up (at the health care provider that works with our HMO) they didn't have it. I searched high and low and discovered it is a formula made up by the Clinic and I could only get it there. Full price, but the prescription got filled. It took about 3 hours out of my afternoon to solve the mystery. We are trying 3 days without milk products to experiment and see if it will impact the diarrhea.

The same drug that is causing his diarrhea has another side effect of shaking. Bob will shake uncontrollably. It is mostly his hands and arms. He hasn't used the iPad since Day 0 and has a lot of trouble with the phone or utensils. Another new happening is his blood vessels are very close to the surface of his skin. One of them just popped and started bleeding. This is because of low platelets. So all of these things are normal and to be expected. They will pass with time or stop when the drugs are stopped.

One of the things that writing the blog did was keep me focused on the future. When I sat down to write, it was my time to summarize the events the best I could. I would try to remain optimistic on issues we were facing. If a topic made the blog, it had to be making a big impact in our lives. One of those events was Bob's diarrhea.

It wasn't an issue that I could give many details about on the blog. Out of respect for Bob and the gross nature of the details, I just mentioned it as one of his biggest issues. It was exhausting for both Bob and me. For Bob, it meant he never knew very far ahead of time if he needed to go. He would have repeated accidents. Sometimes he would be up, but most times he would be in bed and not even know anything had happened. For me, it meant stripping the bed and washing the bedding. I ended up asking housekeeping for two extra sets of sheets. I needed to have clean sheets available at all times. I put towels under the sheets on the bed and on the chair he sat in, for added protection.

I felt like I was constantly running up and down four floors to wash all the bedding and pajamas. I used bleach to clean everything and found myself washing the bathroom with the bleach mixture almost every time it was used. I think on the worst day I changed the bedding four times. I made sure I always carried a change of pants for Bob wherever we went. It was during this stressful and exhaustive time that I met what I refer to as my pad angel.

Bob had checked-in at the infusion room for his daily treatment. We never knew which nurse we would have assigned to us. On that particular day we were greeted by Nurse G, our nurse for the day. She reminded me of pictures I had seen of the nurses during World War II. She had medium-length, curly, gray hair, tan slacks, and a short-sleeved blouse that buttoned up the front. The blouse was white with a small flower print, and the collar was rounded.

I immediately liked Nurse G. She was a no-nonsense kind of gal. She was to the point, but compassionate and caring. Nurse G introduced herself and starting asking Bob questions about how he felt. This was the common routine every time we signed into the infusion room. She was aware that Bob was in his first two weeks of his posttransplant period. There were many details and observations to be aware of.

One of her questions was concerning how often he was going to the bathroom. Bob answered that he had diarrhea every time. She then went right to the question of how much his fluid intake had been. Bob answered, "It's okay." Then she turned to me and asked for specifics. I pulled out my notebook that had all food and fluid intake and read the amounts to her.

She asked Bob some more questions, and then while getting the IV started, she glanced over at me and asked, "How are YOU doing?" I looked up at her and told her the truth. I didn't whine, but just bluntly said I was washing bedding and clothes constantly. In her matter-of-fact and efficient way she finished settling Bob in and then disappeared.

About fifteen minutes later she poked her head into the room. Bob was asleep, and she came over to me and handed me a neatly folded pile of washable pads. She told me they used them in the hospital and at the clinic and that they were wonderful. They were cloth on one side and a washable plastic on the other side.

She handed them to me and said, "These will save you having to wash everything every time. When you are done with them you can drop them in the soiled hamper here at the clinic and they will go through the laundry." I looked up at Nurse G and our eyes met. I couldn't say what I was feeling. All that came out was, "Thank you!" What I was feeling was someone had heard **me**. Someone cared about **my** connection to this exhausting, scary experience. Someone took the time to listen, react, care, and show kindness to someone other than the patient. Nurse G was definitely my angel for that day.

Strength means recognizing that it is impossible to be strong all the time.

Sally Franser

23. Up the Hill

I remember at one of the first meetings when we arrived at the clinic we were asked to fill in a caregiver form. It was a list of all the caregivers' names, relationships to the patient, their phone numbers, and the dates they would be staying with the patient. The patient was not allowed to be without a caregiver at any time.

I didn't think much of it as I put my name down as the sole caregiver. It wasn't until I met others at the housing facility and clinic that I realized the bigger picture. Some patients had family members share the responsibility. Others had friends serve as their caregivers, and there were a few that paid an organization to have someone be their caregiver. It humbled me to see all the patients with their different caregivers.

I never felt like a martyr as Bob's caregiver. I really felt I had a job to do and I always tried to do my best. I knew I would impact Bob's success in his battle by the way I faced the challenges of being his caregiver. There was nothing that could have prepared me for my role of being a caregiver in that stage of his recovery.

There was so much that had to be done that I started each day like a horse coming out of the starting pen at a race. I ended each day so tired that the minute I hit the bed, I fell asleep. I always tried to get up early and go down to ride the bike for thirty minutes. It was a great plan, but I knew it was always just that, a plan. It was one thing I could do for me and yet be following the guidelines of being a caregiver. During the posttransplant, pre-engraftment time that Bob felt so terrible, my role as caregiver was intense and overwhelming. My years of being the hovering helicopter paid off.

I had a special notebook for recording food, protein, and fluid intake. It traveled with me in my backpack. Taped on the counter at the apartment was a form used twice a day to record Bob's temperature and blood pressure. The red binder was by far the most important and most used of all the notebooks and folders I used for organization. It held our daily schedule, special instructions, printouts of blood work, and the four pages of medications that he was taking. This was with me wherever I went. If I was asked a question concerning Bob's care, the answers were in my backpack. Once we got home from the clinic I would empty the backpack and record in the notebooks that evening and repack the bag for the next day.

Bob would go to bed most days when we got home from the clinic, and I would run and do laundry and start dinner. I got very efficient at multitasking. After putting a load of laundry in on the first floor, I would go to the second floor where the kitchen was and start the meal. By the time the laundry was ready to go in the dryer, we were ready to eat.

After eating I would fold the clothes and bring them up to the second floor and finish washing and sterilizing the dishes. Once the dishes were put away I would literally drag the laundry bag up to our apartment on the fourth floor. Most times when I got in the room Bob would have all the lights off and be back in bed. It was such a difficult time for him. He felt lousy with no energy and when he used Hell to describe that period of time, it was accurate.

Every night I filled Bob's pill container for the next day. Many evenings I did this with a small night-light shining above the list of medications. Oh, those medications! I took many deep breaths when it came to the medications.

I was unable to use the clinic's pharmacy to purchase Bob's medications. We were out-of-state and had insurance with an HMO, so we had to use the HMO within the state. The facility was located about two miles from our apartment. The two-mile trip was a steady climb up a very steep hill. Many times I would talk to myself about how happy I was that our car was an automatic and not a manual transmission. It would have been one more challenge I would have had to deal with. I always referred to the trip to go pick up Bob's medication as going up the hill.

In all the times I traveled up the hill, there was not one trip that did not produce stress. In the beginning it was a simple thing, like they hadn't received the fax from the clinic. I solved that by always having Nurse J give me a hard copy of any prescription they faxed in. Service was done with by taking a number. The minimum time I waited for my number to come up was thirty minutes. It usually was forty-five minutes.

One time I needed to call Nurse J to have her clarify something and found there was no cell service in the building. I had to leave the building, make the call, and come back to take a number again. Another visit I arrived, waited for my number to come up, got to the individual booth with my hard copy of the fax and heard the person on the other side of the window say, "Oh, we don't have this drug. We ordered it and it will be here tomorrow." Tomorrow, was she kidding? What if the patient HAD to have it tonight? Why hadn't they called the clinic to let them know? Please, not another up the hill trip!

I always felt the trips up the hill were my practice for patience, peace, and letting go. It didn't help that I was exhausted, emotionally drained, and felt alone. I attacked this challenge by calling on Ruth, my wonderful friend. Every time I got in the car to head up the hill, I would call her. I would start the conversation with, "Hi, Ruth, I'm on my way up the hill!" She would sigh and start me on my deep breathing before I ever arrived at the parking lot. She would keep talking to me as I walked to the building. She also told me after I got the prescription to call her back, if I needed to talk.

The first few times I called her, she recommended I stop for a Green Tea Frappuccino, as that always calmed her nerves. There came a time that I just pretended to call Ruth on my way up the hill. I could imagine her conversation as I drove. Her laughter and words of advice were embedded in my mind and heart. My dear friend had connected with me every single day since we had arrived in May.

When it is dark enough, you can see the stars.

Ralph Waldo Emerson

24. Another Hospital Visit

Tuesday, July 19

I wanted to give you a quick update. During the night on Sunday Bob got a fever of 102. There are instructions what to do for each tenth of a degree of a fever. I called the after hour's number and was connected immediately to the head nurse on the special floor at the hospital that handles transplant patients. After looking up Bob's record on the computer she instructed us to come in. With neutrophils at 0, there was no choice.

Since 4 am on Monday we have found out and are doing the following:

- He has a sore on the inside of his cheek. It was caused from when they pulled his teeth (pre-transplant) and the enamel on one of the remaining teeth was chipped and rough. Since he has retained so much fluid, the swelling of his body (including his cheek) has caused it to rub and cause a raw spot. They are testing the sore for infection, but as of tonight, it looks like there is no infection. The remedy: they formed a mouth guard for him to wear at night and gauze between tooth and cheek during the day. Neutrophils must come up before permanent remedy can be approached.

- He has fluid in both ears. Not sure why, but it is causing discomfort and hearing loss. They are giving him Claritin and Sudafed to help it.

- They have aggressively added and increased his blood pressure medications. It has been high since the transplant. Today, for the first time, it is normal.

- He is now wearing "Ted" stockings for the swollen legs and feet. He likes them and they are helping in his comfort.

- He has fluid in his lower left lung. The only thing we can do is get him up frequently, sit upright in chair, walk to get muscle to move fluid around, and practice opening his lungs with an inhaler. Last night they had to put oxygen on him while he slept as his oxygen level was too low.

We are not sure how long he will have to stay in the hospital. One Doctor said once a transplant patient with zero neutrophils has a fever and is admitted, they don't let them leave until the neutrophils hit 0.5. His were 0.14 today. Maybe he will be an exception. Fingers crossed. I have come back to the apartment both nights to sleep, shower, and get supplies for the new day.

We have learned that this journey changes from minute to minute. It is amazing how the ripple effect occurs over and over. We know this is all part of the process and still feel blessed that Bob is doing as well as he is.

Keep us in your prayers and I will keep you updated as things change.

The period of time spent waiting for engraftment was probably the worst and most agonizing for both of us. For Bob he felt terrible. I do believe emotionally he was experiencing more hope and anticipation than he was fear or depression. He was attentive to all the doctors and nurses and always gave 100 percent effort on any suggestions they made. He accepted my hovering and would often make requests of things he wanted or needed help with.

This window of time for me was exhausting both emotionally and physically. Physically, I was responsible for all Bob's needs. He did shower himself, feed himself, and get dressed on his own. I was responsible to make sure everything was in place for when he needed it. It was overwhelming keeping on top of things.

Months before, during the caregiver class I attended, they stressed the importance of taking the patient's temperature twice a day. That would establish a baseline for a normal temperature for Bob. They also passed out laminated cards to be carried in our wallets with the phone numbers of all their facilities. I remember one of the instructors going through different scenarios and quizzing us on which number would we call.

That practice came to mind as I watched Bob's temperature start to rise. I didn't even comment or tell him what was happening. He was in a restless sleep and my interruptions to take his temperature meant nothing to him. As I watched it go up I referred to the printed sheet of paper that I had taped on to the wall next to the phone. It was explicit on exactly what tenth of degree to call in. It was after midnight, so my communication would not be with the clinic but with the hospital.

For me, this hospital visit was completely different than the first one. Before I even called, I packed my backpack with a change of clothes for myself, chargers for my phone and iPad, pajamas, slippers, and personal items for Bob. I packed all the medications and written information concerning Bob's care. I got dressed and even packed a toothbrush for me and my own blood pressure medicine. Yes, I had changed in the last few weeks. I was much more matter-of-fact about Bob's care. I knew that anything I couldn't or shouldn't handle would be taken over by the clinic, the team, or the hospital. This was one of those times.

I made the call to the hospital, as instructed. The phone call went directly to the floor that deals with transplant patients. The head nurse asked a few questions and looked up Bob's record on the computer. She said, "You will have to bring him in. Our rules are if a posttransplant patient has a fever and neutrophils are 0.0, they must come in." I replied that I understood and asked about parking and getting him up to the eighth floor by myself. She informed me she would alert the night guard, and that I could leave the car in the front circle for up to an hour.

I was extremely calm as I woke Bob up and told him we were going to the hospital. At first he fought me and said, "I'm fine," but he reluctantly agreed after I told him we had no choice because of his temperature. It was a silent drive to the hospital. Not a word was spoken. As we approached the front circle I asked Bob if he was scared. "No," was all I got from him. I reminded him things would be just fine and that we were headed to the best place possible.

The head nurse greeted us and got Bob settled and told me to go ahead and park the car. She recommended a different parking lot, closer to the hospital. I can remember going to the car, in the pitch dark of night, and being calm. I took a deep breath and knew Bob was in good hands and I could relinquish my helicopter hovering while he was in the hospital. I had no fear for Bob. I only had confidence that this too would pass. I remember taking a deep breath of the fresh air and looking up at the stars as I reentered the hospital. The cool air felt good in my lungs, and although I was exhausted a certain peace had come over me.

During the hospital visit I had my own schedule. I went back to the apartment every evening by seven o'clock and arrived back by six thirty. I would purchase a coffee on my way up to the room and get a report on how Bob did during the night from the nurse before the shift change. After the morning doctor's visit I would leave the room and get something to eat.

i was with Bob throughout the day and would record his steps as we walked around the halls, record his food and protein intake, and not worry one bit about his medications! I was aware they were changing, but knew I would get the updated printout when he was discharged. I felt like a pro. I was rested, showered, and alert for communications and interactions.

One of the projects I delved into during that hospital stay was searching the internet for available houses on our favorite island. It took a lot of time and that was something I had plenty of. Bob took many naps and the time was filled with me making notes in one of my numerous notebooks. Bob knew that I was on this new project and would check in every once in a while to see how I was doing. I came up with five possibilities for us to someday go look at. It was something that served as a dream for when this journey got to a place of being a little more predictable.

Out of difficulties grow miracles.

Jean de la Bruyere

25. Good News

Thursday, July 21
Well in two days we have more news.
Bob did have some pneumonia in his left lung.

So....the GOOD/WONDERFUL news! Bob has officially been declared as being successfully engrafted. What that means is the new cells have taken over. We can tell because the neutrophils are multiplying rapidly to a high level.

This is the first cross road that we needed to get to. ALL of his numbers are increasing, but these are the ones that represent engraftment. I had tears in my eyes as I looked at the numbers. Bob is more quiet and reserved. I asked him what he was thinking and he said, "I still have a long road ahead of me with bumps to get over". One of the bumps will include Graft vs Host Disease. This is true, but we are thankful for today's positive news and jump the bumps as we hit them.

Tuesday, August 2,
Hi Everyone,

Today is our wedding anniversary and we celebrated with lunch out after Bob's infusion. We walked the few blocks to a local restaurant and shared a hamburger and fries. We sat outside on a patio in sunny 72 degree weather.

We have several things we are celebrating today:

- Being together for 42 years and still loving/liking each other. The real test of love is living in a dorm setting 24/7 for 5-6 months. We are surviving and still have a sense of humor.

- Blood work today showed numbers stable. His whites and reds are just about the same as last Friday's blood work. Platelets went down just a little.

- Tomorrow marks 3 weeks since his last blood transfusion. He has not gone that long in years. He shows no signs of needing one.

- A Bone Marrow Biopsy has two results. One part shows chromosomes makeup. All results since he was diagnosed have shown MDS in his marrow. Our BIG celebration, and miracle, Friday's bone marrow biopsy results show NO SIGNS OF MDS in his marrow!! None zero, gone!

This has been a very special day for us. We are celebrating today and where we are today in our long journey. The picture is of us at the clinic for his magnesium infusion this morning before all the good results were given to us.

I get by with a little help from my friends.

John Lennon
With A Little Help From My Friends

26. Ruth's Visit

With the wonderful miracle of engraftment, the dark days leading up to it faded in our minds. Both Bob and I continued to focus on the future. Even if the future was just one day, we looked forward. One of the things I looked forward to was visits from friends.

Before committing to any visitors or outings, I checked with other patients, families, staff, and caregivers to see when a reasonable time was for having visitors. Bob had to feel reasonably well and his counts had to be high enough to fight infections. We decided on a date of August 9 for Ruth to fly in. Jackie and Jack made reservations for an August 25 arrival, which would be Day 55. Phil, my hairdresser, would arrive on September 9. In between those visitors would be continued visits from Anastasia and Robert.

One of the realities I soon became aware of was that visitors couldn't stay in the apartment with us. Originally, I had hoped the hide-a-bed would be a good choice for having guests. Early on, Anastasia arrived and stayed with us in the room. We discovered immediately not only did Bob need his privacy, but being in the environment for too long was a high-stress situation for the visitor. Bob went to bed at seven and did not want any noise or lights.

Any television or music was enjoyed with headphones. There was only one pair of headphones, so when Anastasia and I were together, we flipped a coin to see who would get them. No phone conversations were allowed in the room after the lights went out. No lights meant I found myself filling Bob's pill container using a night-light. Anastasia was a trouper and stayed with us whenever she visited. I knew why she went for long walks and why she was always relieved to go home. Her visits were so appreciated by me. She was a needed support, but also in some ways she validated me as I faced the situation on a daily basis.

Once Bob engrafted and the calendar started filling up with visitors, I felt myself relax just a little. My conversations with friends and family were less intense. I talked some about the details of Bob's treatment, but I took time to hear their news, and we shared our excitement of their upcoming visits.

As I reflected on this difficult time, I truly realized and appreciated the miracle of an unconditionally giving friendship. I found that I had a special connection with each friend. I didn't share the same information or emotions with everyone. It was amazing to me how each individual impacted me. It was as if each were a beautifully wrapped gift with a colorful bow on it. I held a special place in my heart for each person. I found I valued each unique relationship and friendship beyond words.

Ruth had not missed one day of checking in with me. It was sometimes just a quick voice message that said, "Thinking of you and hope all is well." Other times she would call and update me on her happenings before I told her the news of the day, after asking, "Is this a good time?" She was definitely living our daily journey with us. She was compassionate, patient, non-judging and above all, a good friend. The journal entry I wrote on the CaringBridge blog did not come close to sharing the details and stress that poor Ruth experienced during her visit.

Wednesday, August 17, Day 47

Since the last update we have had some ups and downs. Bob continued to do well after his bone marrow biopsy. Each day he seemed to be getting stronger and feistier. We had our good friend Ruth visit and give support for a week. She had a room across the hall from us and was able to get a feel of our days, events, health care, favorite restaurants and a general feel for the Pacific Northwest. We so enjoyed our time with her. In the beginning of the visit, Bob was walking ahead of us as we went to the market and on another day he walked with Ruth down a big hill from the clinic to one of our favorite restaurants for lunch. They walked and I brought the car.

It was this energy and good spirit that led us to think we were well on our way. Saturday morning Bob woke up and just didn't feel right and stayed in bed to rest. We assumed he had been moving and going quite a bit and needed a day off. By Saturday evening he had a fever and by 9:00 pm the three of us were on our way to the hospital. We had to follow the procedure when his temperature reaches a certain mark. They gave him a chest x-ray, blood work, and an antibiotic and sent us home because his white counts were high enough that he was not neutropenic. Sunday they called from the clinic and wanted to see him and he ended up 5 hours at the clinic. No fever during the day.

Today he is much better. I think the antibiotic is hitting anything that might be in there. The tweaks that the doctors do daily to his regiment are watched closely and evaluated. We do not feel alone. We have wonderful and amazing care with such compassionate professionals. We are in good hands.

I share this with you to represent the change from wonderful to fear and unknown within one day. Sometimes the change can occur within 15 seconds. You cannot plan ahead of time for anything as circumstances change at record speed. The glitch we are coming out of was a sign from above to take a deep breath and live this moment with no plans or expectations for tomorrow, next week or next month. We are not out of the woods yet.

What was missing from the update on CaringBridge was the extreme minute-to-minute stress that went on during Ruth's visit. We both enjoy plays, and we had committed to a Sunday matinee of *Les Miserables*. It was a big commitment to purchase three tickets ahead of time with the hope that Bob could make the performance. Ruth and I had also committed to a cooking class, one block away from our apartment. The cooking class would take us through making the complete dinner and end with the class sitting down to enjoy the dinner. The whole adventure was from six to nine on the Saturday evening before the play. How perfect. Bob usually was in bed by seven, and we would be home, relaxed, and fully satisfied from an elegant, gourmet dinner. What could go wrong?

Making those plans with Ruth so far out from her visit was exciting. I felt like I was going to be normal again. Having fun with a friend, planning activities, and having Bob at a point where plans could be made felt good. I convinced myself that this was the turning point for my stress level to return to a lower intensity. The visit did start out busy, as I had shared on the blog. Ruth stuck with us like glue. She participated in every infusion, doctor's visit, washing and folding of clothes, and making of meals.

She experienced the new stubbornness that Bob displayed. He walked ahead of us wherever we went. He rarely asked either of us where we wanted to go or what we wanted do; he just started out doing it, and we followed. At the time I think Ruth and I felt happy that he had such determination and energy. His feistiness was different from the pre-transplant Bob. In another time it could have been labeled as rudeness. Ruth and I would wander off and take walks whenever Bob was napping. It seemed like we always ended up sitting with a couple of Green Tea Frappuccinos. I knew they made her happy. I should have realized they served as a stress releaser for her.

Sometime in the middle of her visit, I shared with Ruth our thoughts about maybe buying a house on our favorite island. The reason was to stay close to the support of the clinic, but also because the surroundings were amazing. She was in shock. Bob and I had thought about this for months and never shared it with anyone. I knew everyone would think we had lost our minds to be considering such a big decision in the middle of a life crisis. I knew how it sounded, but I also knew the comfort and peacefulness that came with the support and expertise of those surrounding us. Ruth was quiet and reserved for the entire evening. By morning she reacted with the solid support of an unconditional friend. She said, "If this is what will make you happy and is best for you, I am behind it."

The blog never mentioned that Saturday's plan was to drive north to the island and show Ruth the favorite house we had picked out. Bob felt exhausted, so he stayed behind and Ruth and I drove the hour north. In the car Ruth talked more about us moving and what an impact it would have on her. She promised not to mention the possibility to anyone else. She respected that it was something I wanted to share face-to-face. It never dawned on me that asking this favor added one more weight to her already heavy stress load.

Ruth loved everything about the island and house. She fell in love with the 180-degree views, the fact the house was one level, and even the spacious bathrooms. She was excited for us, and as we drove back to the apartment we discussed ways I would break the news to my mom, family, and friends.

When we arrived back to the apartment, Bob was still in bed. I immediately felt panic and guilt. I had left him alone, and he was running a temperature. We had two hours before the cooking class. I insisted she go. Our payment was nonrefundable and it would be a new adventure for her. I ran down the hall to one of the caregivers I had become friends with to see if she would like to go in my place. She was excited for the opportunity to be participating in a fun activity that had no connection to caregiving.

It took a lot of convincing to get Ruth to go. She made me promise that I would call her the minute Bob's temperature reached the mark where I would have to take him in. I promised. At 9:15 PM

I called and told her I was going to take him to the hospital. I asked, "How's the dinner going? Have you eaten yet? Can they pack you a box to go?" She was anxious and stressed, I could tell. "No, we are still cooking! I don't think we will eat before ten. Can you pick me up in front of the store?"

Ruth experienced the entire minute-to-minute stress of the unknown during a hospital visit. The stress was impacted by the lateness, the tests that needed to be run, the waiting, and the nervousness of not knowing. By one thirty that morning we were on our way back to the apartment. Bob's white blood cell counts were high enough that it was safer away from the hospital.

The next day was Sunday. Our matinee performance was at one o'clock. At ten in morning we received a call from the clinic informing us that they needed to see Bob to check him out. Off to the clinic we all went. I knew by eleven thirty that I was not going to make it to the play. They hooked Bob up to receive several different infusions. The timeline to release him was about five o'clock. The nurse encouraged me to go. He would be fine. I hesitated for several minutes and then decided to go.

We asked Maria if she would like to come with us and use Bob's ticket. With my phone on vibrate, the three of us settled into our seats and the music began. I had a strange tingle in my body as I looked around at the audience and observed all their faces. They represented a normal, fun activity that I hadn't experienced in such a long time. The performance took me away from all the stress of the last four months. I squeezed Ruth's hand and said, "Thank you for being here with me."

At intermission I went into hovering mode and started getting anxious. I figured out the performance would end close to five o'clock and with twenty minutes added on to get out of the parking lot, I decided to leave at four. Maria decided to stay, and Ruth and I snuck out and hit the road. Bob was just finishing up when we arrived at the clinic.

I delivered Ruth to the airport and got the call she arrived safely. The news that she went into the hospital upon her return impacted me. She had severe heart palpitations and felt as if she was having a heart attack. Was it all the stress she had experienced during the visit? Was it all the stress of Bob and the news of us moving that led to the Green Tea Frappuccinos, which then led to the heart palpitations? The answer would not be found.

Ruth's visit awakened me to several emotions and observations that were buried inside me, just out of reach.

- I missed the familiarity of friends and family.
- I missed the life outside of the clinic and caregiving.
- I was aware that Bob's attitude and response to those around him was abrupt, isolated, and at times rude.
- I appreciated and cherished my friends.
- I needed more hugs than I was getting.

While we may not be able
to control all that happens to us,
we can control what happens inside us.

Benjamin Franklin

27. Nervous Breakdown

The weeks following Ruth's visit represented a change in me as the caregiver. Bob became stronger and stronger. Along with his renewed physical strength came a feistiness that I had not seen in a long time. When I looked at the big picture I was thankful for each day and accepted each change in Bob with the attitude, "It is what it is, and I am lucky to have him here." Down deep, I was glad to have him alive, sharing each day together. Down deeper there were other emotions surfacing.

I remember feeling used. Really used and not appreciated. Here it was August and Day 50 out from the transplant, and I was just churning with emotions of feeling used. I felt sorry for myself that I did everything from cooking, cleaning, laundry, meds, organizing, and chauffeuring without one squeeze, hug, or a check (I love you) from Bob.

I knew the trigger for these emotions was a combination of the recent visit with Ruth, being able to see and share with a good friend, and also having Bob become more independent and not need me as much. It was a formula for hurt feelings, and I knew I was very emotional.

As Bob felt stronger, we started to walk the eight blocks to the clinic. We would start out together, me with the backpack, my purse, and any other supplies for the day. Within a few blocks, Bob would be way ahead of me with never a glance over his shoulder to see how I was doing.

I observed he would come to a corner and never slow down or glance to see if there was traffic coming. He would step off the curb and plow forward. At the apartment, he would be demanding and blunt about needing laundry done or food prepared. I think if I had been at a different place, I would have recognized his independence, stubbornness, and bluntness as the result of a person who was no longer at death's door. It was the result of a person feeling the freedom and power of having some control back in his life.

I remember lying next to Bob one night and starting the conversation with, "I need more attention from you. I need to know you appreciate me." This was not the first time in our forty-two years together that Bob had received the talk. I always had been outspoken and blurted out my feelings. He lay there quietly and just let me blab on and on.

About five minutes into my teary-eyed speech, he spoke up and said, "So, what I hear is that you need a hug." So far there had not been a hug, a squeeze of my hand, or a word of appreciation. I sat up in bed and looked at him and yelled, "If this was a movie the audience would be booing you! They would be yelling for you to just give me a hug!" I lay back down on the pillow with sniffles and a clogged head from crying. He put his arm under my head and pulled me to his shoulder. We both fell asleep with no more words being spoken.

The next day I overhead Bob talking on the phone with Robert, saying, "I don't know what is wrong with her. I think she is having a nervous breakdown. I think you should come and get her and let her stay with you for a while." As I listened, I covered my mouth so he wouldn't hear me laugh. He was clueless. His focus was how **he** was feeling, and at this point, he was feeling great! It was so out of character for me not to be calm and collected, he didn't know what to say or do.

Robert called me within five minutes of hanging up with his dad. "Mom, what is going on? Are you okay? Why don't you come up and stay with me for a vacation and get away?" The conversation brought me to my senses very quickly. My answer was, "No, that is not possible. Thank you for the offer, but someone has to be with Dad, 24-7. Besides, coming up to your confusion would **not** be a vacation to me." I assured him that I was fine and would work it out. It was at that moment that I realized the reality of my situation.

One of the concepts that had proved to be most helpful to me was my awareness and acknowledgement of my realities and expectations. I recognized the realities in my life and tried to keep them close to 100 percent. I did the same with my expectations, but tried to keep them as close to 0 percent as possible. I found this formula worked for me to help keep my life more level without drama and disappointment. I had daily practice with this formula as I participated in my role as caregiver, mom, daughter, and sister.

I remember talking to Ruth the night I overheard Bob tell Robert that he thought I was having a nervous breakdown. I told her that I knew my complaining about not receiving attention might be viewed as a nervous breakdown to others, too. She reminded me of the Rs and Es formula. (Reality and Expectations) We'd had many conversations in the past about practicing that concept.

It was like a lightbulb turning on. I immediately realized the reality of situation. The reality was that Bob was not going to be mushy or sensitive to my needs all of a sudden. He was where he was, and I needed to accept that. It didn't change the fact that I needed acknowledgement or a hug. By expecting it from him, I elevated the disappointment that came with expectations.

The next day we had an appointment with the doctor. We were sitting in the examination room as Nurse J took Bob's vitals. I randomly asked her if there was someone I could talk to. She responded with, "What is the issue you would like to discuss?" I replied, "I just have some emotions that I need to vent." She continued, "Well, yes, we can get you an appointment." She turned to Bob and calmly asked if he had any issues and he replied, "No, everything is just fine with me. She is the one that is all upset."

Nurse J kept busy with the tasks at hand, but kept the conversation going. She glanced over at me and said, "Do you feel like you have been thrown to the curb?" I just nodded my head up and down. I was afraid I would cry if I spoke. She then turned to Bob and gently reminded him how much it takes to be a caregiver and that I was one of the best around.

Nurse J made arrangements for me to talk with a social worker the next day. The appointment was scheduled during one of Bob's infusions, so it worked out very well. I had a nice conversation with her and was able to vent quite a bit. It wasn't just venting, but while I shared my feelings and thoughts, I felt I was sorting through everything.

She talked about what Bob's point of view might be, now that he knew he would survive and had a life ahead of him. Now that hope was in his vocabulary again, and he felt like he had some control again. It all made sense to me. I knew it was up to me to accept and/or get past the feelings of being used and not appreciated.

I wondered if other caregivers had similar feelings. I left the meeting with the social worker feeling calmer and quieter. I would work on my Rs and Es and maybe open up some conversations with the other caregivers at the apartment.

There is no distance too far between friends,
for friendship gives wings to the heart.

Author Unknown

28. A Visit with Dear Friends

Monday, August 29, Day 59

Your kind words, warm thoughts and constant prayers are all appreciated and accepted with a smile. I hope your all know how much your positive energy has meant to us. We feel the support and love from all of you.

We are back on track on Day 59 already. We don't look at the calendar like we use to and when someone asks us what Day we are on we have to think before answering.

Our dear friends, Jackie and Jack, came for 5 days. I just got back from taking them to the airport and feel very sad but happy to have had the special time with them. The time flew by and we squeezed so much into their visit. Lots of hugs and then some more hugs. We have a tradition of sangrias so I made some and we pretended to be on our back patio looking at the Rocky Mountains.

We wish you all a fun and safe Labor Day Weekend! It was one year ago on Labor Day we flew out here for our consult. Who could have guessed we would be here one year later with the Transplant completed!

There was so much that I couldn't share on the blog. Our visit from Jackie and Jack was even more emotional than Ruth's. They arrived and settled into their apartment across the hall from us. Jackie and I prepared a favorite meal down at the community kitchen. Bob acted antsy and abrupt during dinner. Jackie said the area was beautiful and asked if we liked it. Bob just blurted out, "We love it and are going to move here!" I saw the shock and surprise in Jackie's face. She was in shock.

When Bob was done eating he just got up and left. I knew he was done for the evening. He was shutting down. He never spoke any common courtesies to Jackie and Jack like, "It is good to see you, but I am really tired and think I will go to bed." No, he just got up and left. I could read Jack's expression. He was in shock. I wanted to cry. Not only had Bob's behavior been rude, but he spilled the news about moving without any thought or care to their feelings.

I sat with them and told them that we were seriously thinking about moving, but had not done anything about selling our home or buying another. All the pros and cons were being considered. Jackie's reaction was exactly why I had wanted to tell our friends and my mother in person. This was the kind of news that needed hugs and eye contact when shared.

Jackie and Jack spent the entire next day glued to every appointment and happening that was on our schedule. Since Jackie was a retired nurse, she was very interested in the clinic and the care Bob was receiving. As we all sat with Bob during his infusion time, Jackie abruptly got up and left. After about five minutes I left to find her. She was in the bathroom, and I could hear her crying. I knocked on the door and asked her if she was alright. A soft-spoken yes was the only response I got. I stayed in the hall waiting for her for about twenty minutes.

When she opened the door I knew this whole encounter was extremely emotional for her. The news that we were thinking of moving, seeing Bob in the surroundings of his medical care, and experiencing everything in real life versus hearing about it on the phone was overwhelming. I put my arm around her shoulder and squeezed. There were few words I could speak that would make her feel better. She apologized and said she would be all right. I knew in my heart that this hurt was deep and that it wouldn't be all right.

Jackie and Jack did a little sightseeing on their own, and I took them to a few places while Bob rested. We decided to ride up to the island and see if we could get in to see our first-choice house. That seemed to perk Jackie up a little, and going through the house with its beautiful view brought a smile to her face. We even kidded about which bedroom would be theirs when they came to visit. We ended the trip by sharing sangrias on the deck of the facility where our apartment was. There had been many hugs and tears.

My plan was to fly back home during Labor Day weekend. I had three days to stage the house, put it on the market, and, the hardest thing of all, to break the news to my mother.

A real decision is measured
by the fact that you've taken a new action.
If there's no action, you haven't truly decided.

Tony Robbins
Awaken the Giant Within

29. Labor Day Weekend

Once we made the decision to move, the first action had to be to put our house on the market. Bob was doing well but still needed a caregiver 24-7. I called Anastasia and asked her if she could come from Friday night until Tuesday. I planned on flying out on Saturday morning and being back early afternoon on Tuesday. She had already used up her sick days by coming to be with Bob and I previously. Without hesitation she said, "Mom, I'll work it out. I'll be there."

Both Anastasia and Robert responded to the notion of us moving very calmly. I think the fact that the house near the Rocky Mountains represented our retirement home, not the home they grew up in, made it easier for them to accept us selling it. They had no emotional ties to it. Anastasia was concerned about doing it during the posttransplant period of time. Bob's energy level was better but still limited. I felt the importance of acting sooner than later. I knew being close to the clinic as Bob faced the first year after transplant would be a gigantic advantage in his well-being. After all, they knew him. They knew his history, and from my perspective they had become like family.

So with Bob's care covered by Anastasia, and his pills in individual compartments labeled by day, I set off for the airport. This was the first time I had been away from Bob in months. I felt strange and awkward. My thoughts on the plane were of Bob and where he was in this journey. Yes, he was doing well and improving with each day. After nine years of living moment to moment, I couldn't help but wonder about the what ifs. What if he had a setback or worse didn't make it? How would I feel being so far away from family and friends? Was I strong enough to take care of selling the house and buying a new one by myself? Was I strong enough at this stage of my caregiving to take on this mammoth plan of action? What if we moved and Bob didn't make it? I made the decision on the plane not to play what if with the future. We were moving forward with our decision.

I had decided not to let my mother know I was coming in until after I cleaned and staged the house. The only people who knew I was coming home were Ruth, Jackie, and Jack. I knew once I connected with family I would want to be near them and spend time catching up and hugging. There was also the reconnection to Angel. Would she remember me? I was nervous about breaking her pattern for just three days. The poor girl would be so confused and frustrated. No, I would see Mother, Angel, and family after the house was officially done.

When I say I came home to stage the house, I mean that it needed to be cleaned, uncluttered, and ready to list. The house had seen much activity since we had left it the previous May. My brother Charles had lived there for two months, and later Robert had moved in and stayed until August.

It was strange walking back into the house. When I entered I had to catch my breath. There were many emotions bottled up, and they all came out with that first breath. There was the immediate emotion that this was home, but strangely it represented our old home. Another emotion I felt was this house was enormous compared to our current 450 square-foot apartment home. The surge of all the memories made in the house flowed through me in that single instant. As I let out that first breath I felt the tears collecting in my eyes.

After walking through the entire house, I started making a plan of what had to be done. Our Realtor, Dave, would come by Monday night for me to sign the papers and take some pictures for the listing. The For Sale sign would go out on Wednesday morning.

There was so much to accomplish before Monday evening. I went to work on bagging extra items that I would eventually sell at a garage sale or donate. The bags included linens, stuffed animals, knick-knacks, framed pictures, and just stuff. The bags ended up in the basement storage area with a large sheet covering them.

Next, I attacked the cleaning: washing floors, shining appliances, and placing furniture just right. By Sunday evening I had just about completed everything, so I made the call to my brother Charles. I asked him if he would come over to the house and bring mother with him. He wanted to know why I was home and asked if everything was all right. I told him Bob was good, and I would tell them everything when they arrived.

My mother is an amazing soul. She had tears in her eyes as we hugged and her first question was, "Is Bob okay?" Over a cup of coffee, I told them the story and reasons for putting the house on the market and moving. I could see the pain in my mother's eyes, but her words were supportive. "I had an inkling that you were going to move! You love the area and love the care Bob is getting." She was sad, but at the same time I could tell she was supportive and happy for us.

Dave arrived Monday evening with all the paperwork and his camera. Bob and I had decided to list the house for fifty-five thousand dollars more than Dave had recommended. He gave us a price that he thought would help sell the house quickly. After all, the housing market had bottomed out. After signing the papers, a flood of exhaustion fell over me. I had been going nonstop since I stepped off the plane on Saturday afternoon. I had visited with Ruth and Jackie and Jack. I had spent time with Angel and many of my family members. The amount of physical and emotional energy used in those three days had drained me, and my tank was on empty.

I walked through the house one last time before leaving to catch the flight back to Bob and my responsibilities as his caregiver. I spoke out loud to the house as I walked room to room. "You are a good house, you have good bones. You need a family with children and lots of activity." Sitting on the plane and waiting for takeoff, I looked up to the sky and whispered, "It's in your hands."

I had written an entry for our CaringBridge blog before I left to put the house on the market. Bob posted it Monday evening once the papers had been signed and it was official.

Monday, September 5

We wanted to update all of you on our happenings and our special news.

First, Bob is doing wonderfully. It is Day 66 and he is still getting great reports from the doctors. The final result of the Bone Marrow Biopsy is not in, but the first results showed no sign of MDS.

We have had a life changing journey while here. It has impacted us in a way we have never experienced before. We have a chance for life that 8 months ago was only a hope. We have looked at each other and asked what we would like to do with this gift of additional time.

We have decided to make the leap and live our dream. As of today our house in Colorado is on the market. We have found an Island we love. It is about an hour north of Seattle. We feel that this move allows us to be close to excellent health care, close to our children and of course, we LOVE this area of the country. I know this will sound crazy, risky and just plain nuts but trust us we are sure of the decision. If the house sells, then we know it was meant to be.

We feel sad thinking about being so far from friends and family. This process will take time which gives us time to come back to Colorado and spend some special time with everyone. For those of you that have lived the last 9 years with Bob and me, you realize the joy that we have in our hearts knowing we have more precious time to celebrate live with each other and our children.

All is grace.
Nothing happens by chance.
Everything happens for a reason.

Joel Randymar

30. Speechless

I was truly exhausted when I returned to Bob and the apartment. I flew back on Tuesday following Labor Day weekend, and Anastasia left for home on the same day. Tuesday night I prepared Bob's pills for the next day, got all the notebooks in order, and ran some laundry through. I hit the pillow that night so tired that I had no energy to worry about the house selling or not. I really had given it up to be what it was going to be.

The next day we found ourselves at the clinic with more infusions. We were in good spirits as we knew the For Sale sign had been placed out in front of our home that morning. Dave, our Realtor, told us we would be called each time someone had an appointment to go through the house.

Being the efficient list-making person I was, I told Bob I would keep track of all the showings and see how many we had. The first call came about eleven thirty that morning and the Realtor on the other end said the house was being shown at one o'clock. Bob and I just smiled, and I entered the agency, date, and time of showing in my notebook. We felt we were off to a great start. I think the nurses and team members thought we were just a little nuts acting on our decision to move to the area. Bob was still a long way from being discharged. After all it was only Day 68. He would not be considered to be discharged until Day 100, and that was only if all went well. We knew all the facts, but again, the house might not even sell.

We arrived back to the apartment by one, and Bob had lain down for a nap. The phone call came at three. It was Dave, and he started the conversation with, "If you were going to be in town, I think I would like to hire you as my official house stager." I laughed and thanked him before asking, "How did the showing go?" Dave replied, "I mean it--IF you were going to live here, I would hire you to stage houses, but you won't be living here. You have a full-price offer on the table from the first couple that went through!" I was speechless. "Are you kidding me?" I finally sputtered out.

He reassured me it was for real. The couple had been living and looking in the area for months and had another offer on a house fall through. They were living in temporary housing and wanted to move. "Could you do a late September closing? Oh, and one more thing, the couple is from the Seattle area." It was like a dream. I knew a September closing wasn't going to be possible, as Day 100 was on October 9. I told Dave I would get back to him right away so he could get the offer in our hands by that night. Wow! A full-price offer! Bob and I couldn't believe it. We had our signal from above that this move was meant to be.

The paperwork was sent to us electronically, and we signed it with all the dates in place. The closing on the house would be October 18. That would give us nine days to get back to our old home, pack, load the truck, see family and friends, and oh yes, try to have all those last-minute doctor appointments before changing our health insurance. Our heads were spinning.

The next day, with the signed document in our hands, we immediately called our Realtors (Keri and her father, Don) up on the island and told them we would like to put an offer on our first-choice house. They were surprised, but thrilled, to hear we had sold our house so quickly. Bob had done some research on the property value on the island and houses that had recently sold. We decided on a price and wrote an offer and by Thursday night it was in the hands of the owners.

On Friday morning my friend and former hair-dresser, Phil, arrived for a planned five-day visit. He wanted to support us and visit us when Bob was feeling well enough to have visitors. Phil was a genuine, compassionate, and fun friend. His sense of humor was one of a kind and his compassion was sincere and appreciated. As with all our guests, I arranged for a room across the hall from us. He settled in and joined us at the clinic, where Bob was receiving his daily infusions. We showed him around the clinic, and he helped me prepare dinner in the shared kitchen. Phil is a wonderful cook. Friday night at dinner we heard back from Keri and Don that the owners of our first-choice house would not budge. Not one dollar. I guess our offer was an insult. We figured we had room to play, as it had been on the market for three years. Not so. No counteroffer.

We were disappointed, but Bob was firm in his belief that the house was not worth much more than we offered. I was okay with the decision to not counteroffer, as I knew we would find another house. We asked Phil if he would like to drive up to the island with us the next day and look around, and maybe we could get the Realtor to get us in to see our second-choice house.

So we all settled in for the ride on Saturday. Phil was interested in seeing where we would be living, and he was happy that we wanted and respected his opinion. We arrived at the house, and while sitting out in front of the house waiting for Don to arrive, Phil commented, "I am not feeling this neighborhood. I just can't see you here." We went through the house and I had to agree with Phil. We all agreed. Bob and I sat down at the kitchen table and started talking about possibly renting a house and storing our belongings until the right house came on the market. All of the homes we had looked at were smaller than our Colorado home. We were thinking about downsizing and trying to get a house that was one level.

Bob mentioned to Don once he arrived that we could afford a bigger home, but just thought we would downsize. At that point he looked at us and said, "I just passed a house on the way over here that recently went back on the market. I'm not sure what the history of it is, but I noticed it is getting a new roof put on it. It is similar to this one, but I think bigger. I have never been through it, but would you like to try and go through it since you are here?" We all looked at each other and I spoke up first with excitement and said, "Why not?"

We followed Don for less than a mile and pulled up to a stunning property. There were men on the roof and in the yard, and there was a buzz of activity. I couldn't believe that we were going to go through this gorgeous house. The foyer opened up to windows that showed a 180-degree view of water. The colors in the house were done with such wonderful taste. Don walked with us through the house, but because he hadn't been in the house he did not know details of its history. Bob and Don sat in the main room discussing the price of the house while Phil and I took in every detail. We discussed colors, flooring, woodwork, fireplaces, and the gardens, and sometime later met up with Bob and Don.

It seemed the reason I had not looked at this house while surfing on the internet was because it was not in our price range. Bob asked what the price was that had been accepted before and decided to offer well below that number. Don, bless him, never flinched. He said he would verbally tell the owner's Realtor about the offer and see where it went. It was **so** low.

As we filed into the car and headed back to the city, Phil, Bob, and I just kept talking about the beauty and details of the house. Before we reached the apartment, Don called and told us that the owner said if we would come up a small amount and not debate the inspection (the last inspection produced a new roof) that he would accept our offer. That was Saturday night about five o'clock. The next day, while Bob was in the clinic getting infusions, Phil and I went to work on copying the paperwork and faxing it. By noon on Sunday we had all the paperwork signed and in place.

Then we waited. Phil was due to leave on Tuesday morning. We all had different ideas on if we would get the house. Phil was the only one that was confident enough that he insisted we go out Monday night and start celebrating as we waited for the call. The later it got that night, the more nervous I became. Finally, at seven the phone call came. The house was ours. In six days' time, we had sold our home and purchased another one.

As the events of the week sunk in, I really reflected on how blessed we were. I reflected on the miracles that had happened. The feeling I kept coming back to was grace. It is easy to recognize but really hard to describe. I felt in harmony with everything around me. I felt there was a reason why everything had happened. I felt at peace that we were in the arms of angels and being guided. I felt divine love. I felt that the universe had just hugged us.

Every exit is an entry somewhere else.

Tom Stoppard

31. Exit

Signing the papers for selling a house and buying a new one turned out to be the easy part. There was so much to follow through on. Thank goodness we had great Realtors representing us on both the sale of our old home and the purchase of the new one. It seemed a day did not go by that the phone would ring and bring another decision to make concerning inspections, appraisals, loans, or details of paper-work. I felt the added stress as I lay in bed at night.

For some reason I wasn't quite as focused on how many grams of protein Bob had consumed in a day. Bob was focusing more and more on all the details of closing on the houses. I was impressed at the amount of energy he had. He began to view the infusions and doctor appointments as the wall between him and leaving the clinic. He started asking the Red Team questions about the chances of a patient ever being released early. I found myself reflecting on the previous months and how there were times after the transplant that I pondered about Bob's survival. There we were, not only surviving, but looking to a future that included major changes.

The day Phil flew home was Day 74 for Bob. He was antsy and less compliant with all the recommendations made by the team. His common response to me was "I know! I know!" followed by him doing what he wanted to do. I found I treated his attitude with a big sigh and chalked it up to him living for so long with no energy, choices, or control of the smallest things in his life. In fact, I was grateful that he wanted to be more independent.

I found myself reflecting back to how it was before the MDS diagnosis. During that time Bob would handle his things, and I handled my things, and, we hardly ever walked on each other's turf. As the journey had progressed to the present we had no division of duties or turf. The turf had become a gravel road, and I felt like it was up to me to travel it pretty much alone. So I accepted his new attitude with gratitude and hope of a new beginning.

Our days were still full with visits to the clinic. Bob received a magnesium infusion daily, and it seemed the blood draws were more frequent. We were so focused on our exit (the term used in meetings for us leaving) that it didn't occur to us that the team was in the process of a massive checklist. All of the tests that Bob had completed before the transplant took place had to be revisited. The impact on his body of the actual transplant and the massive amount of drugs he was consuming had to be evaluated before any talk of an exit could be discussed.

For a solid week and a half, our calendar and schedule was completely full. In addition to the daily magnesium and occasional hydration infusions and blood draws we now were busy with many other appointments. We traveled off campus to visit a cardiologist and a kidney specialist. Bob revisited radiology and pulmonary testing, saw a nutritionist, and even had a successful dentist exam with confidence.

We attended an Orientation Class on Day 96. It was called that because the nurse that held the class would be helping all those in the room to orientate themselves back into the real world ... the world outside of the clinic. We were very excited going into the class. To us it represented being closer to our exit. We received a letter to give to our family and friends that explained his restrictions. Pictures were shown of patients that had Graft-versus-host disease (GVHD).

We had met a few patients that were diagnosed with GVHD. GVHD occurs if the new stem cells do not recognize the organs and thus try to get rid of them. GVHD represents the delicate balance of the new cells taking over and the old allowing it. If not watched and monitored, it can be very serious. The reality of the information presented put a damper on our excitement. It was clear that Bob was not out of the woods and could still encounter extreme challenges.

As we plowed through all the appointments and tests, I found a curious change occurring in myself. As I traveled back and forth between our apartment and the clinic, I thought about how I would miss the familiarity of this place we called home. One might think I would want to run from it as fast as I could. Not so. I found myself hesitating at the cafeteria line and asking the chef how his mother was doing with her move. I stopped and talked with the person on duty at the desk at our apartment complex. I had been friendly and supportive with other patients and their families at the apartment, but now I wanted to pause just a little longer to talk.

I found myself in the waiting room for the blood draw, looking around at all the people and at their eyes or color of their skin and wondering where they were in their treatment. My heart was filled with compassion and support for them. This was a far cry from how I felt during my first visit to the oncology waiting room, back when Bob was first diagnosed so many years ago. I was completely out of myself and into the room. I was not standing on the outside thinking I didn't belong, but instead I was standing with them as part of the family we were. I realized the growth and compassion I felt was the daily fuel I needed to refill my internal tank.

Late in the afternoon on Day 97, we arrived for a summary conference. I brought the list of all Bob's medications and together we sat across from Nurse J and our Red Team doctors. The summary included a very formally typed report about Bob from the day he was diagnosed eight years earlier. It included all the good, bad, and ugly facts about his treatments and responses to them. The sentence that was amazing to me was that he no longer had MDS. There was no MDS! Bob asked one of the doctors if he was cured. The doctor answered, "Yes, we can say you are cured of MDS, which means you will not die from MDS." There were tears in my eyes as I listened to the report and looked around the room at all of us. That group of people represented so many others that all had worked together to come to the point in time where Bob was cured.

The next day Bob had the Hickman line removed from under his skin. The pulling of the Hickman represented a freedom from the daily infusions and flushing of the lines. I felt as if the umbilical cord had been cut. We flew out the next day (Day 99) to return to our Rocky Mountain home. The closing on our home was in ten days. We had completed our exit successfully without any fears or thoughts of where our new entry would take us.

If you know you're going home,
the journey is never too hard.

Angela Wood
Judaism for Today

32. This Way Home

We arrived back at our home in Colorado with days to complete all the tasks involved with selling, closing, and packing up a house. Each day was filled to the brim with things to do. Once again, Bob had his list and I had mine. We wanted to include special time with family and friends. The movers needed two days to pack the house and another day to pack the truck. It was a whirlwind of activity, which left little time to step back and wonder about our decision to make this big change in our lives. The days were filled with much physical and emotional exertion. By the time we got on the airplane to fly back to Washington State, my body was numb and my eyes were puffy from all the good-bye tears.

We had decided to fly versus drive, as the closing on our new house on the island was two days later. We left Angel with my mother with the plan that my brothers, Charles and Tracy, Mom, and Angel would drive our second car out three weeks later. The plan was that it would serve as a vacation for them once they got there. It also gave us a little time to start unpacking and try to get guest bedrooms ready.

Ruth offered to come out and help me unpack, and I accepted her offer. She arrived three days after the movers had neatly deposited the many boxes in their designated rooms. I made sure she had a put-together bedroom and bathroom when she arrived. I don't think Ruth could have been prepared for the enormous task ahead of her. She cheerfully asked what I would like to attack during her short week visit. We mutually decided that getting the kitchen in order was a priority. After four days of unpacking dishes, Ruth repeated several times, "I see a completely new side of you!" Every time we opened another box of china, she would repeat the question, "Where did you have all this stuff at your old house?"

I always had the tendency to approach most tasks in my life with the force of a hurricane and an effort of rarely less than 100 percent. This approach was evident in all I did including cooking, gardening, scrapbooking, and even in being a mother, wife, friend, and caregiver. Unpacking a house was no exception. We had moved several times in our lives and unpacking was something I had always done pretty much on my own.

This time things seemed different. I was older. I was tired. I had gained some wisdom about what really counted. On the third day of unpacking, I glanced up and looked at Ruth and saw in her face the same tired and worn-out feeling I felt throughout my body. What a trouper. She was going to hang in there as long as I kept putting a box in front of her. I smiled and said, "This is the last box we are doing. We are going to have some fun and relax before you have to go home."

The next day Bob, Ruth, and I ventured out to locate a talked-about small town that was rumored to have quaint shopping and yummy restaurants. We enjoyed the day together with each of us making a special purchase. Ruth found a great top, Bob bought a rain coat for Angel, and I purchased a sweatshirt for Bob. It had "LIFE IS GOOD" printed across the front of it. When I saw it, I knew it summed up how we felt about our lives. We felt blessed to be out doing normal things, breathing fresh air, having energy, and most of all being alive.

Ruth's trip ended with us relaxing another day, taking in a movie, and finding another new restaurant for dinner. She repeated to me several times how happy she was for us. Every time Bob would get tools out to help me hang a picture or as he began to unpack the office, Ruth would comment and remind me how well he was doing. She had been with us through many years of stress and struggle.

Unpacking continued slowly. By the time Mom, Angel, Charles, and Tracy arrived, we were ready for guests. Bob was in a routine of doing small projects around the house in-between his biweekly visits to the oncologist. Thanksgiving brought Robert and Anastasia home, and as we sat around the Thanksgiving table we were all thinking the very same thought. How thankful we were. It had been a long road with many bumps and rough patches, but we were here. We were together. We were home.

Anger is nothing more than an outward expression of hurt, fear and frustration.

Dr. Phil McGraw

33. Frustration and Anger

Thanksgiving came and went, along with all the company. Things quieted down with a comfortable routine evolving. We dug into repairs and got to know the details of the house. There was a wood-burning fireplace in the family room that Bob fell in love with. With a stack of firewood left behind, he enjoyed the fire nightly. We had a big propane tank on the side of the house, which fueled the other fireplaces, the cooking range, the water heater, and the emergency generator. We figured out what had to be done most of the time by accident. One day as I was cooking the flame went out on the stove ,and I fidgeted with the knobs and finally yelled to Bob for help. He checked the outside propane tank and realized we had run out. With an emergency delivery that afternoon we learned the basics about timing, supply, and demand.

We were traveling the hour to the clinic about every three weeks to visit the Long Term Care Follow Up team (LTFU). The local oncologist, Doctor J, who had been referred to us by the clinic, was a more frequent visit. He was a wonderful doctor who greeted us each time with a smile and was truly interested in Bob's posttransplant journey. Bob would have blood work on the morning he visited and go over the numbers with the doctor during his visit. They would discuss Bob's energy level and activities he was doing.

On the morning of December 5, before his doctor's appointment, Bob was wrapped in a towel brushing his teeth, and I glanced over and saw redness all over his skin. At first, I thought it was from being in a hot shower. I went over to have a closer look and saw hundreds of small red dots. "How long have you had this rash?" I asked Bob. I had the same feeling I'd had the day I discovered the infected cyst a year before. Bob nonchalantly replied, "It has been there a few days, and it is nothing to worry about." All the way to the doctor's office, I was beating myself up. Why hadn't I seen this? I felt I had let up on my hovering and look what happened!

Doctor J gave his opinion about the rash. He believed it was Graft-versus-host disease (GVHD). He took pictures of Bob's skin and sent it on to the clinic. He would get back to us. GVHD is common for posttransplant patients. It is the battle of the cells. The old cells just don't want to give up their space. In the fight that goes on the new cells attack the host body. The common parts of the body that show signs of the attack are skin, eyes, and mouth. The important part of the struggle was to control the attack so it stayed in check and didn't attack or impact vital organs. We knew about GVHD. We had seen pictures during the exit class in August of what GVHD could look like. Were we being naïve to think it was not something to be concerned about? The reality was we had been in our own life is good world with the shades pulled down to any more health issues.

Within days we heard from Doctor J and the LTFU at the clinic. They wanted to see Bob as soon as possible. As we made the hour trip to the clinic, we both verbalized how happy we were to be so close to experienced, caring professionals. As we drove by our old apartment and parked at the clinic garage, I had the overwhelming feeling of peace. I was home and help was right through the front door. I knew they would know exactly what to do. I had another feeling flowing through me. I was back on as caregiver. I had my calendar, notepad, medical records, and list of medications. Yup, I was in hovering mode.

The common treatments for GVHD are immune-suppressing drugs. A common one used is Prednisone. I had never heard of it, but was confident the team knew what they were doing, and I dutifully took the prescription and wrote notes, including the next appointment date. Bob was to take sixty milligrams daily. They told us that he might not be able to sleep well at night and that he might gain weight, as the drug makes people hungry. For some reason, maybe because I just wanted someone else to be in charge or maybe it was my complete trust in our doctors, I never Google-searched the drug Prednisone.

By Christmas, a few weeks later, I had noticed a few subtle changes in Bob. He was eating much more. He didn't want to sit at the table with me to eat, but preferred sitting in his chair and eating while watching television. He didn't like what I cooked. He started buying his own food, consisting of frozen burgers, desserts, and pretty much whatever he wanted.

He was obsessed with having the fire burning most of his waking time. I felt it was the medicine and couldn't stop my caregiver mode of worrying about him. It was after Christmas dinner when Bob blurted out, "Will you all be quiet! I can't hear the TV!" that I knew Bob was changing. Robert kept defending his dad saying, "He survived and is alive … let him be." I had to agree with Robert, but somewhere deep down I knew that the Bob I knew was fading and disappearing. I also knew the patterns of our relationship we had shared for forty-four years were gone.

I was wise enough to know that I needed to be doing more than caregiving for Bob and running the house. I needed to interact with others. I needed to get out of the house more than delivering Bob to a doctor's office. I started to look into organizations that I might enjoy being part of. I decided to visit a meeting of the local branch of the American Association of University Women (AAUW). I sat at the meeting with a feeling similar to what I experienced sitting at the production of *Les Miserables* with Ruth five months earlier.

I was more interested in observing the interaction between the other women than listening to the guest speaker. I recognized the nonchalant and giddy conversations between them. It was so obvious to me that I lacked that in my life. I missed being relaxed and chitchatting about non-life-threatening issues. I joined AAUW that evening with hope and new energy. Little did I realize that I would not attend another AAUW meeting during the upcoming year.

It was during this time of searching and needing interactions with others that I started speaking to a neighbor across the street. Ed worked in his yard a lot, and I could tell he took great pride in his work. I would comment on his lawn, and one time I asked his secret for not having moles in his yard. It had not taken me long to realize everyone had a secret to rid their yard of these pesky rodents.

I felt like Bill Murray in the movie *Groundhog Day*. I had tried gum, hair, poison pellets, and liquid detergent. I made up my mind I was done trying the day the poison worm I had placed deep down the hole was sticking out of the top of the mound the next morning with not a nibble taken out of it! Ed was eager to share his solution. He brought all his special tools and taught me basically how to tend to the mounds so the lawn would not be ruined. It was a great solution. The moles were still moving around underground, but the lawn didn't have the mounds all over it. It was after Ed's mole lesson that I mentioned we would like to have him and his wife over for dinner. Did they like salmon? It was settled. I would call his wife, Patty, and set the time and date.

Inviting neighbors for dinner made me happy. I felt so normal again. I had always loved entertaining. I set the dining room table and planned a great dinner. We all had a glass of wine before dinner. Patty and I chatted while I was busy with preparing the meal, and Ed and Bob were in the family room.

I didn't notice Bob had opened another bottle of wine. By the time we sat down to dinner, Bob was in rare form. He did not eat very much of the dinner. During dessert he started talking about our sex life, in detail, back when we were first married. This was something Bob hadn't discussed between us in forty-four years, much less with neighbors we were just meeting for the first time. I could feel the warmth rising to my face. What was going on? I had seen Bob tipsy before, but this was much more. There were no boundaries. I quickly closed the evening with, "Bob really should have only had one drink tonight. Mixing alcohol with his medication is a no-no."

Within ten minutes Ed and Patty left and I started clearing the dishes and cleaning red wine spots from the carpet around Bob's chair. I was upset. The evening was not what I had planned. I was embarrassed. The very first time getting together with the neighbors and Bob talked detailed sex?

I heard a loud noise in the back of the house and went running. Bob had fallen and was on the laundry room floor laughing. There was blood all over the floor, door, and his arm. He had ripped his now-thin skin as he fell. After getting Bob cleaned up and in bed, I returned to the kitchen to clean up dinner dishes. At another time in our lives, I would have looked at the incident and seen the humor in it but that night I was angry, embarrassed, and petrified that my life as I knew it was over.

The next morning I sat on the ottoman facing Bob. That was my favorite place to be when I wanted him to hear and see me. I asked him what he remembered about the night before. He replied, "Not much." I asked him, "Would you like to know what went on?" I think he knew I would probably tell him anyway, so he said, "Sure." I relived the night before with all the gory details. Included were my emotions of being scared when I saw the blood, and feeling alone, embarrassed, and angry.

After that, I left the house and started driving. I didn't have anywhere to go. I ended up at Bed Bath & Beyond, buying new sheets to replace the bloody ones from the night before. I sat in the parking lot and talked to Anastasia for about forty minutes. She was a good listener, but this time I picked up on something that I hadn't felt before. As I shared the story, I got the distinct feeling that she didn't think it was as serious as I did.

I felt the glimmer of her being tired of hearing constant stuff about her dad. Did she think I was making too much of things? Did she understand my perspective? Did she realize how difficult and frustrating it was to cope with living with someone who covered his ears whenever you spoke? I made up my mind that day that I would not burden friends and family by sharing my frustration and anger. I would begin to tell fewer details and complain less not only to Anastasia and Robert, but also to Mom, Ruth, Jackie, and anyone else that checked in.

When you reach the end of your rope,
tie a knot in it and hang on.

Thomas Jefferson

34. Hanging on by a Thread

The Prednisone period was the darkest time I had ever faced. It was about losing the man I had been with for forty-four years. The Bob I knew and loved was MIA. Some of the despair I felt came about from being alone and isolated. The depression that engulfed me was mixed with anger. Some of the incidents were daily and represented a gradual change. Other happenings were such traumatic events that I felt I was living in a movie. I chose to think of it as a comedy versus a horror film. If I laughed, it seemed a little like make-believe.

One such incident that felt like I was in a bad dream was while picking up a headboard I had ordered for our bed. I was excited about finding a great deal and felt from the measurements we could get it in our 4Runner. We drove the thirty miles to pick it up at Tuesday Morning. When we tried to load it into the car, I realized it was never going to make it.

Bob was agitated and went in the store, yelling at the young clerk about not having any materials available to tie it on. I suggested we find a neighbor with a truck and see if we could get help later to pick it up. Nope, not going to happen. Bob sped off and found a hardware store and bought a paring knife and some rope. He put the headboard on top of the car and ran the string around it and got in the car to go. I stood outside the car and said, "This isn't going to make it." He responded with a blunt, "You do it and tell me when you're ready to go."

This may not seem so horrible to some, but for me it was devastating. This was the man who for all our married years had to do it all. He knew best. He was in control. The consequence of him doing it all was that I became dependent on him and lacked confidence to attempt his things. I had taken on much more since his diagnosis, but he had always been there to support me. He was now living in a cocoon. He was oblivious and without care to me and those around him.

I stood outside the car and ran the rope both vertically and horizontally many times. I stepped back and thought that I probably should run the rope around the headboard and through the windows of the back seat. I had the plan I would sit in the backseat and hold the rope tight. The whole time I was wrapping rope, Bob sat in the driver's seat with the door wide open and the radio on full blast. He had shut me and the world out. I felt the tears coming to my eyes as I wove the rope over and under.

I was angry, frustrated, and felt sorry for myself. I finally started looking around at the people walking by, and I focused on a gentleman in his 50s. I approached him and asked him for his opinion. "Do you think this will make the drive on I-5 for twenty-five minutes?" He walked around the car and leaned over and looked at Bob and then came around to me. "Who is that in the car?" he asked. I told him it was my husband and added, "He is not himself. He is on some strong medication." He walked around the car and tightened the rope in a few places and recommended we not go over forty-five miles per hour.

As I sat in the backseat with my hands pulling down on the rope, I remember saying a prayer asking to get us home safely. About fifteen minutes down the road Bob asked if I was hungry. I said, "NO, let's just go straight home." Within a few minutes he exited and drove up into the parking lot of a casino and asked, "Are you coming?" I said I didn't feel comfortable leaving the headboard on top of the car. He didn't hear my response as he was on his way to the buffet. I sat there thinking I was in a dream. This didn't just happen. As I looked down at the blisters on the palms of my hands, I knew it was real.

I knew I needed to do something for my own sanity. I decided to book a flight back to Colorado and get away. I arranged to have an open house at my mom's for all my friends to stop in. I wrote everyone an email, letting them know the time and date, and ended the message with, "I coming back for some hugs." I knew what I needed. The visit was wonderful. I got hugs, conversations, smiles, laughs, and rest. I returned after five days with my mother by my side. I had invited her for a visit. I was bringing normal back with me. I knew I would have someone who would have a conversation with me and not cover her ears when I talked.

During my mother's visit another serious incident occurred. This incident had to do with the fireplace. Bob loved having a fire. It made him happy. One night I was at the other end of the house and I smelled smoke. I assumed Bob and Mom were together watching television. I rushed into the family room to find the fireplace door wide open with wood on the marble mantle burning and black smoke bellowing out. "What's going on?" I asked. Mom was on the couch in shock. Bob was sitting in his chair while on the phone with Robert and replied, "It got too hot so I opened the door and the wood fell out."

I was yelling by then, "Why are you on the phone? Help me take care of it!" He continued on with his conversation with Robert and said, "Mom is ragging on me. Wait a minute, I am going to move." With that he got up and left the room. Several things at this point were completely out of character for Bob. First of all, to have an open fire in the house would never have happened before. His pride of caring for things and common sense were always in place. Secondly, Bob would never have sat and talked on the phone as a crisis evolved. He would have stepped up and taken control. Thirdly, he had **never** spoken about me the way he did to Robert.

Knowing it was up to me to solve the problem, I immediately started with trying to get the burning wood back into the fireplace. Even with gloves on and using tools, I burned my arms and singed my hair and eyebrows. I continued the cleanup process by washing all the black off the bricks on the fireplace with soapy water. I cried during the whole cleanup. I felt anger at Bob's response. I had difficulty catching my breath. I would look back and realize the anxiety attack I was experiencing at the time was a warning sign. As I turned off the lights in the family room, I took inventory of the damage done. The marble in front of the fireplace was melted down several layers. The rug in front of the fireplace had several spots and holes where the sparks had landed. How lucky we were that I hadn't had to call the fire department.

The next morning I knew I had to talk to Bob about what happened. The marble and carpet could be fixed. I was more upset and worried about the lack of safety and common sense. He responded to our conversation with, "Don't worry, there is no more firewood. Last night I used just kindling wood and that's why it got so hot." He said he would fix the holes in the carpet. I made a plan to buy a big area rug and put it in front of the fireplace. A few days later as I dropped Mom off at the airport, I reflected on feeling validated having her there to experience the change in Bob.

I found myself sticking very close to the house. Bob had done several things that scared me. He made lunch for himself once, and when I walked in I smelled fire. He had burned the pan beyond repair and set off the fire alarm. He repeatedly went through stop signs, and when I asked him, "What were you thinking?" he responded with, "There were no cars coming." These were things that constantly had me thinking of not only his safety but mine as well.

A few days after Mom left, I attended a lecture on pruning held at a local community center. I knew I would only be gone a few hours, and Bob promised to call if he needed me. When I arrived home and walked into the family room, I had to sit down and take a deep breath. In a very calm, quiet voice I asked Bob, "What are you doing?" He was on his hands and knees and had cut out, using a paring knife, a four- by three-foot piece of the carpet located in front of the fireplace. He had proceeded to lay a piece of carpet he had found in the basement into the hole he cut out. The edges were raveled and the seams did not match. He was in the process of taking ashes out of the fireplace and throwing them over the new section of carpet and rubbing them in.

I was in shock. Was this really happening? I went and got my camera and started taking pictures. As I took pictures I asked Bob, "So can you explain why you are putting ashes on the carpet?" Still on his hands and knees he replied, "I am making the new carpet look old to match better." I left the house with Angel to take a walk. I stopped and called Robert and told him what had just happened. I wasn't crying and told the story as if it was a scene from a comedy movie. The truth was I was in shock. "Any suggestions?" I asked Robert. He said, "Geez, Mom, I don't know what to tell you. It is so unlike Dad. You know it is the medicine. Just keep an eye on him so he doesn't hurt himself." I hung up, realizing our future was in my hands.

Bob had only been on Prednisone for three months. There was no discussion or mention of when they would take him off of it. Without Bob being my partner and not having family and friends close by made daily living such an effort. The Bob I knew and loved was nowhere to be found. I was now his enemy. I grew angrier with him. I found myself reacting before he would talk. I stayed away from him as much as possible. I was literally at the end of my rope.

I think that when you invite people to your home, you invite them to yourself.

Oprah Winfrey

35. The Tulip Visit

A weeklong visit from three good friends from Colorado had been planned for three months. Jackie, Sharan, and Nancy had chosen mid-April as the time for their visit. The local area celebrated a Tulip Festival during this time. As the time came closer for their visit, I felt my level of anxiety rise as I thought of their visit with Bob in the house. His behavior and attitude were unpredictable. I phoned Anastasia and asked if her dad could spend six days with her in California. She agreed and the flight reservations were made.

The preparation for the girls' visit was my joy and sanity. I made out a calendar and researched places to show them and restaurants to visit. The four of us had celebrated our birthdays together, and I had missed a year of celebrations. I made gift bags for each one of them and included carefully selected items. I included passes to see a performance of *South Pacific*, which was playing locally. I picked a special restaurant that overlooked the San Juan Islands for our birthday lunch and made reservations. Menus for the week were thought-out and planned for. Sangrias were a must to include.

I was a great guide and showed them the area, including walks on the beach. There was an evening spent wrapped in blankets out by the fire pit sipping on sangrias. There were fresh tulips in each of their bedrooms. We included shopping every time we left the house. The highlight of the week was the tulip fields. While we were standing and looking out at the massive, beautifully colored fields, a rainbow appeared against the partly cloudy sky. As I took in the beauty I had tears in my eyes. I took the presence of the rainbow as a special gift just for me. It was a message saying all was well and all would be okay. It was a very surreal feeling. I felt I was the only one in that field looking at the scene and soaking in the message.

The tulip week was magnificent! I felt normal for the first time in over a year. During the visit I had shared my feelings of anxiety, loneliness, and frustration. I told the girls I felt like Bob was losing me. At the time I didn't think too much about what emotions the girls were going through as they observed me in my current state. They knew me as a positive, hopeful, and compassionate person. The person they saw and listened to during their week-long stay was not anyone that they recognized. Nancy shared that she felt I was very angry. Her honesty and openness was appreciated. At times I was short and curt with my answers and comments with the girls. I showed signs of much stress. Their entire visit was so needed. I would never be able to say the words to express my gratitude toward the girls for their visit.

A few weeks after their visit, Jackie wrote me an email. I knew I had hurt her feelings with a comment I had made during the visit. I had called and apologized and then gave her some space. The email was short and to the point: "After thinking about this I have come to the conclusion that some friendships are for a reason, a season or forever. I believe ours was for a reason. The reason was to be there while Bob had MDS. Now that he no longer has MDS Jack and I feel it is time to move on. We wish you and Bob the best in life." And that was it. My phone calls and emails were not responded to. That email was the last time I communicated with Jackie.

It goes without saying the email was devastating to me. It was like a death, and I mourned the loss. The event impacted me tremendously. I had lived the majority of my life believing that everything happened for a reason. This event was going to be very difficult to reason with and accept. I found myself looking in the mirror and facing the fact I had been venting and stressing with friends and family for over ten years. Some had traveled the entire

MDS journey with Bob and me. Had the stress and venting been too much? I made a decision and commitment that I would acknowledge each and every person in my life that had supported me during this journey. I would say thank you and express my gratitude. I was on a mission to thank as many of these special people as possible.

I thanked Ruth every time we talked for being the friend she was. She was steadfast, calm, and supportive. She was my anchor in the storm. I repeatedly told her how much I valued her friendship. During my conversations with Sharan and Nancy after the tulip week, I reminded them how thankful I was for their support and honesty.

Judy, my sister who has MS, was someone that I called whenever I feared losing Bob. One might think I would not want to talk about death with a person that faced it head-on. That is exactly why she was the one I called. She spoke freely of her feelings, and when I hung up from talking she always left me in higher spirits, knowing that each day was special.

Phil had been my hairdresser before we became friends. Phil's concern and compassion encompassed me as the caregiver and Bob as the patient. He reached out with sincere, honest friendship. I realized how fortunate I was to have Phil in our lives.

Minda was a person that connected with me every month or so. She was twenty years my junior and had been in our lives for over twenty years. I met her when she was dating the brother of Anastasia's high school boyfriend. Bob and I attending her wedding, vacationed with her, and had supported her through her divorce. She was a super friend. Even though I was old enough to be her mother, I felt more like an older sister. Her advice and patience was so appreciated.

My mother and I talked on the phone almost every day. During our conversations I told her again, like I did every time we talked, "I love you." She knew how special she was to me.

Anastasia was so supportive of me, and I tried to verbalize my appreciation as often as possible. She had said yes to coming to cover for me at the clinic when I flew back to put the house on the market and yes to having her dad during the tulip week. I couldn't remember how many times she heard me complain about her dad. She would always listen and gently drop a thought-provoking observation. I listened to her and appreciated her honesty.

There was one friend that I felt I needed to mend some fence with. This was Rita. Rita and Dan had been in our lives since Anastasia was in tenth grade. Anastasia dated their son for seven years. We shared dinners, a graduation party for the kids, vacations, smiles, and tears. During the transplant, I would call Rita and talk and talk. She asked questions, and at the time I felt we were on the same page. After we sold and bought our house on the island, our communication had dissolved. There had been no Christmas card or communication for three months. I made the decision that whatever was going on, I needed to reach out and be a true friend. Rita shared her hurts and through emails and telephone conversations, we went forward. I was able to reconnect with her and remind her how special she was to me.

Acknowledging my friends and family and focusing on who was in my life served as a small piece of therapy to help deal with the loss of Jackie. I found myself dealing with my emotions on a day-to-day basis. As hard as I tried to be positive and full of hope, I realized I had very little energy left to deal with Bob and life. It took everything I had to get through each day. My breaking point was near.

But I get a little worried sometimes
When I start to lose
Tired of holding it together
When I know I'm going to blow another fuse
I'm at my breaking point
At my breaking point
Well you're never gonna get it
If you don't get up and try
Try and spread those wings around me
Honey let me see you fly

Eric Clapton
Breaking Point

36. Breaking Point

The pattern we evolved into represented a couple that was married but separate. Bob would eat, play on his iPad, and watch the television all at the same time in his overstuffed chair. I would retreat to the other side of the house and found myself sitting on the deck off our bedroom. It was peaceful and my favorite place. We had two Adirondack chairs and a table out there, and I would wrap myself in a blanket and watch the sky as the sun went down over the water. It was my refuge and special place. It was my place to take a deep breath and relax.

After sitting on the back porch and reflecting, I would feel a sense of renewed spirit and hope. Hope that all of my sadness, loneliness, and frustration would fade. I had hope that Bob would miraculously be done with his GVHD, and Prednisone would be a drug in our past. Hope that my husband would return.

One evening after watching the sun disappear behind the hills and sink into the horizon, I snuggled into bed. It was after eleven o'clock, and Bob had not come to bed yet. This was not his normal pattern, but I assumed he was watching a program or maybe he had fallen asleep in his chair. I thought I would take advantage of the quiet and lie there by myself. We were still sharing the same bed, even though there were many circumstances that would have driven many others out of the bedroom. Prednisone and GVHD had coupled to cause many rippled effects on poor Bob. He now snored. I mean SNORED. Even Angel wouldn't sleep on the bed with us anymore.

An issue that was common, and we didn't know why it happened was his diarrhea. It was common for him to start to get up to go to the bathroom and never make it. I would have to clean it up immediately. There were many times in the middle of the night that he would have an accident in the bed. Bob would turn on a clock near the bed that had choices for soothing sleeping noises. In our pre-transplant life, we would have the ocean waves on softly to remind us of Kauai. Bob now would have them playing at nearly the highest level possible, and I felt like a tsunami was about to hit. If I asked him to turn it down, he would cuss at me and tell me to sleep somewhere else.

Again, this was not my Bob. Why, one might ask, didn't I just move into another bedroom? I am not sure why I didn't. I did try a few nights when I was really angry or frustrated, but I believe in my heart I didn't want that pattern to begin. To me it represented me giving up. Of course, at the time I didn't realize the lack of sleep was only adding to the whole picture of my lack of health and well-being.

On that particular evening as I lay there alone, I pondered on why he wasn't in bed yet. I lay there thinking of all the possibilities, and all of a sudden I sat up and bolted for the family room. I had the fear that he might be drinking. I knew mixing alcohol while on his medication was such a disaster. I really preferred him not to drink anything. To date there are only a few things that can trigger me into an anxiety attack. One is Bob having alcohol and the other is Bob having diarrhea. I think it is a little Post-Traumatic Stress Disorder from all the episodes and emotions of me dealing with them previously.

As I rounded the corner of the kitchen, I could smell the Scotch. Bob was trying to get up from his chair and was wobbly. I walked over and took his arm and asked, "What are you doing?" "Having a couple drinks," he slurred. I could feel the anger and heat move up my chest to my face. I could tell from the bottle on the counter that it was more than a couple. I knew I was yelling but was unaware of what words were coming out. He pulled his arm away from me and started walking through the kitchen hallway. He slammed against the counter, tried to catch himself, and hit his arm and shoulder as he went down. I immediately saw blood coming through his pajamas.

There was a lot of blood, and I wasn't sure where he had hurt himself. Was it his thin skin again or did he need stitches? He got up on his own, and I heard myself still yelling words running together coming from my mouth, "blood, trying to kill yourself, you make me crazy." He stumbled up and said, "I'm just fine. Leave me alone." I followed him down the hallway and about ten steps later he passed out and slumped to the floor. At that point I really was most worried about his injuries. I needed to get the pajamas off so I could see if I needed to call 911. The other emotions that came in a close second were fear and anger. I was so upset. How could he do this to me? I started dragging him down to the bedroom. I couldn't do it. I sat down next to him and cried.

Within a few minutes he woke up, and I hoisted him onto my shoulder and guided him to the bedroom. I grabbed an old sheet and laid it on the bed so the sheets wouldn't get ruined from the blood and placed him down. I yelled, "Do not move! I will get a washcloth and find out where the blood is coming from." I ran into the laundry room to get some cloths and returned to find him wrapping himself in the pillows and blankets. They were full of blood. I lost it. I ripped his pajama top off without unbuttoning it and saw that most of the blood was coming from his arm. There appeared to be no cut or gash. All I could see was a five-inch tear in the skin.

Good, maybe that meant no need to call 911. I went back to the laundry room to rinse the cloth, and I heard a big thump and then BANG! It was followed by Bob groaning. I ran into the bedroom to find him lodged between the bed and the glass nightstand--stuck. There was a streak of blood on the wall that went all the way down to his head, and blood dripped down his head and neck. Bob wasn't moving, but he let out a groan every so often.

I freaked out. I pulled him up and yelled some more. On top of his head was a spot the size of a silver dollar that was bleeding profusely. I held the cloth on it to see if there was a cut and realized he had actually hit the wall and scraped a section of skin off his head and had left it on the wall. I was thankful he had not hit the edge of the nightstand or broken the glass and cut himself.

By the time I got him on the bed again, he was pretty well spent. He fell asleep, and I surveyed the damage. He didn't need stitches, his wounds would heal, I would make another trip to Bed Bath & Beyond for another new set of sheets, and cleanup could take place the next day. He and the bedroom would survive. I was not so sure about myself. I found myself shaking from my hands to my knees. I had to sit on the edge of the tub to catch my breath. I walked around the house, trying to take deep breaths, and realized that while I was calm, I needed to talk to someone. I called Robert and Anastasia and left messages to please call me as soon as possible.

It was eleven thirty at night and they were both probably in bed. I was not going to sleep. My eyes were wide open and my heart was racing. I decided to at least wash the wall where his skin and blood were. As I looked over at Bob with the cloth wrapped around his head, I realized if he tried to get up to go to the bathroom there was a chance he could fall and hurt himself again. I knew I was in for a long night.

A little after midnight, Robert called me back. "What's going on, Mom? Is everything okay?" I walked down to the family room and sat on the couch in the dark and told him the story. Robert's first response was, "Geez, Mom, I can't come down. I have a meeting in the morning I can't miss." I was calm and resolved and answered, "I wasn't calling to be rescued. I just wanted to talk and have someone listen." He got it, and we chatted a few more minutes.

About fifteen minutes into the phone call I heard a noise that sounded like an explosion and a rush of water. I jumped up, turned the kitchen lights on, and caught my breath. There was a surge of water flowing from under the kitchen sink onto the floor.

I hung up the phone and ran to check under the kitchen sink. The water softener container had popped off and the water was flowing out. The hardwood floors were covered with two inches of water, and I knew I had to stop the flow. I found the shut-off valve and ran to get all the towels I could find. I used plastic bags to put the towels in when they got too wet. I worked about forty minutes on cleaning up the mess. "What was the worst that could happen?" I asked myself. We might need a new floor if the wood got warped. What would have happened if I hadn't been sitting in the family room in the middle of the night and heard it when it happened?

I walked back into the bedroom and changed the bloody cloth on Bob's head. I was wide awake, calm, but very shook up. I slid my body down against the wall and sat on the floor with the wall supporting my back. I was in the dark, staring at the bed and the calamity that was in front of me. I reflected on the events of the evening and began to talk to myself.

You need to get things in order. You have to stop calling the kids. You can't keep telling people how bad it is. To them it isn't that bad. Everyone is starting to think it is you. YOU are the one that is in trouble, not Bob. The more you talk about it the more it appears the problem is with you. I hate him. I hate what he has turned into. How did I get here? Geez, if I had a gun I would have shot one of us tonight.

I was trying to be funny and lighthearted when I said the last statement to myself. It was the next day that I realized the seriousness of where I was emotionally, physically, and spiritually.

I sat in the same spot all night. I never moved, and I did not sleep. Bob never moved a muscle the entire night. I found out later that in addition to the Scotch, he had consumed he also had taken his Trazodone, a medication for sleeping. I reflected on where I was and came up with a plan.

I had been writing a book about my journey through Bob's diagnosis and treatment. I found it helped me sort through my feelings and emotions. It was therapeutic and validating to be able to verbalize my experience. I realized while sitting on the floor of the bedroom that the life I was living was more stressful than the story I was telling in the book.

I made up my mind that I would box up my book and notes and shelve it. I would know when it was the right time to start writing again. I felt relieved and at peace about my decision to stop writing. I also found myself shocked and scared about the gun comment I made to myself. It wasn't humorous but a sign of where I was emotionally. It really scared me.

The next morning the phone rang while I was in the scrapbook room packing the book away. I did not recognize the Colorado-based number. I answered it and a voice I didn't recognize said, "Chérie? Is this Chérie from Pilates? This is Kathy." I had to think where and when was the last time I was in a Pilates class. Two years ago? This was the Pilates instructor from years before the transplant.

She continued on, "I had a strong feeling this morning that I was supposed to call you. I mean a really strong feeling. It took me hunting all over for a phone number, and this is all I could find. Are you okay? When I get these feelings about someone I know I have to check in with them." As she was talking, with tears in my eyes, I realized the randomness of her connecting with me. Her feeling she had was not random. She was another angel being sent to me to remind me I was loved. We never spoke again after that morning phone call.

A ray of sunshine, a balmy breeze
Are a gift from God above,
And He also gives us faithful friends
To warm our hearts with love.

Author Unknown

37. Rays of Sunshine

I took each day a little slower following the all-night episode. I found myself repeatedly saying, "What's the worst that could happen?" I started to realize that almost all things in the house could be fixed. I continued to work in the garden, mow the lawn, and escape to my back porch to take deep breaths. I was physically exhausted. My knees were acting up again, and my back and sciatic nerve hurt most of the time.

One day while reading the local paper, I saw an advertisement about a Caregiver Class to be held at the local community center. It would run for six weeks, one day a week, and a commitment must be made to attend all the classes. I called to find out more and committed. It was really a class of learning and sharing. Its format was concise and clear. There were rules for sharing, and I felt it was handled extremely well. Most that attended were caregivers for Alzheimer's or dementia patients. I left class the first day realizing that most of these caregivers were never going to get their loved one back from where they were. It was a rude awakening for me as I still held the hope that Bob would return when the Prednisone was withdrawn.

Ruth had another visit with us set on the calendar. This was a vacation trip. There would be no unpacking of boxes. She arrived a month and a half after the tulip week. She discovered both Bob and I were at a different juncture than the life is good place, back in October. It was June and the Prednisone time had been in full swing for six months. She had heard the gory details many times over the phone. I was surprised she wanted to visit. How relaxing could it be, between my stress and anxiety and Bob's unpredictable behavior?

During her visit we decided to visit the King Tut Exhibition in Seattle. I bought tickets online, and the three of us ventured off in the car for the hour trip. Bob was driving, I was the navigator in the passenger seat, and Ruth settled into the backseat. I was always anxious when Bob drove. His vision was not what it was before the transplant, and his multitasking skills were not sharp. There had been the incidents of running stop signs and changing lanes in traffic with cars honking. I found myself being not only the navigator but a backseat driver as well.

We arrived at the parking lot safely and started the spiraling climb up the levels, looking for a spot. Once parked Bob left us and wandered off into the building. Ruth and I paid for parking at a machine and eventually found Bob wandering. We picked up our tickets and made our way to the long line of those waiting to enter the exhibition. Ruth and I told Bob we would just be a minute, and we found a restroom and returned to find no Bob. After waiting fifteen minutes we looked at each other and questioned if he might have gone in without us. I voted yes. We decided to enter with the next group of twenty people and search for him on the inside. Eventually, we caught up to Bob. He was thoroughly enjoying the exhibit and hadn't thought about where Ruth and I were. Ruth commented that he was in his own world.

We arrived back to our car, and I offered to drive. Bob bluntly said, "NO! I will drive." As he backed out of the parking space, I heard a bump and yelled, "Stop! You're going to hit that car." He continued to back out and I could see the car next to us move. As he pulled farther out, I opened the car door to get out and see if there was any damage. I got back into the car, and Bob pulled away and said, "I did not touch that car. You're crazy." I turned and looked at Ruth in the backseat, and her eyes were as big as saucers. She mouthed to me, "Was there damage?" I replied, "I didn't see any." We made our way to the main street on our way to our favorite seafood restaurant on a lake nearby.

Bob continued to drive recklessly by going through a red light and entering a parking lot the wrong way on a one-way entrance. The curve in the entrance was not possible to maneuver, as he was going the wrong way. He stopped and jimmied the car back and forth, trying to get out of the entrance curve. With each forward or reverse move, he would bump the front and then the back of the car bumpers. From inside the car we could hear metal-on-cement scraping each time he made an attempt to go backward or forward. I covered my eyes with my hands. I remember thinking, "What is the worst that can happen?" I knew I needed to get the keys away from him as soon as possible. I could hear Ruth gasping and felt her hand holding tight on the seat.

Bob finally pulled into a parking spot, and I asked for the keys before he opened the door. He refused. He slammed the door and took off on foot to the nearest parking box to pay for our parking. Ruth and I just sat in the car. She started talking very quickly, "Did he REALLY not think he hit that car in the parking structure? How much damage do you think he did to your car? You HAVE to get the keys away from him. He can't drive home!" I was in shock and also nervous about our safety. We walked around the car and surveyed the scratches and dents. It was bad.

As we looked up to find Bob, we saw a line of several people waiting at the parking payment box. They were looking at their watches and frustrated. At the head of the line was Bob with his credit card out saying, "This machine is broken. It isn't working." Bob left the line and started walking over to us, and we observed the next in line having success with the box. Ruth looked at me and asked, "Do I have your permission to ask him to give the keys to you?" I told her, "Please, try. Maybe he will do it for you."

Ruth and Bob came back to the car with Ruth's arm hooked in Bob's arm. Ruth handed me the parking ticket for the windshield of the car, and Bob handed me the keys. Later she told me that she asked him to do it for her and told him that she didn't feel safe in the car. She had clarified that he did hit the car in parking garage, and his judgment was not up to par.

Thank God for Ruth. I sat at the restaurant knowing what a good friend she was. This was supposed to be a vacation for her and she was right in the middle of our new normal. I drove home that day and upon walking into the house, without any discussions, I gathered all the car keys and hid them. The next time Bob went to drive somewhere, he was livid. He knew what I had done. He got in my face and called me a nasty name and demanded the keys. I gave no emotion, no anger, no argument. I simply replied, "NO."

Ruth stayed a week. The three of us went to movies and dinners and took walks. It was the first time since December with Bob starting Prednisone that someone, other than my mother, had stayed for more than a day or so with Bob in the house. Ruth saw the complete picture. I was a wreck, and Bob had changed. She shared her concerns and focused on trying to get me help with the household chores.

Ruth is amazing with spreadsheets and offered to help me set up one with all the tasks done around the house, and maybe make a column for Bob and one for me. We could check off a task every time we did one. I believe she thought he would come to his senses when he visually saw how much I was doing and how little he was doing. She also discussed my trying anxiety medicine for the times I couldn't breathe. I heard her words, but the same thought kept coming to my mind, "Does she think I am the one with the problem? Does she think I am losing it?" As Ruth packed to go home I hated to see her go. She was a friend that had brought a ray of sunshine into my life for a short week.

Phil also had planned a visit with us, and it occurred shortly after Ruth went home. He had not been to the house since the day we had all looked at it with the Realtor. He was amazed at how settled we were and how wonderful everything fit in. Phil immediately picked up on the tension between Bob and me. He picked up on how tired I was, both physically and mentally.

I found him up early one morning out in the yard weeding. He observed that I was doing the entire yard and it was just too much. He went out in the garden with me and helped. The whole time we were working he was talking and listening. "Why don't you try to hire help? You are wearing yourself out." Our discussion floated over to the subject of my anxiety. He highly recommended I see a doctor and get something prescribed to help calm me. He also recommended, as Ruth had, that I make some kind of a checklist with the daily chores listed. He encouraged me to include everything, even the smallest item.

Before Phil left, he wrote Bob a letter. It was a five-page, handwritten, from-the-heart, honest observation. Phil shared with me why he was writing it. He hoped his honesty would impact Bob in some way. Bob gave me permission to read the letter. It was a heartfelt, loving correspondence. Phil shared his own struggle, with depression and how he recognized it in Bob. He tried to explain to Bob how special I was. "All she needs is an 'I Love You' or a hug once in a while. If you don't want to work out in the garden, then sit with her while she is working. It will bring her joy." Phil's honesty was that of a friend sharing his love and compassion with us. He touched me forever with his kindness and tenderness.

Change has a considerable psychological impact on the human mind.

To the fearful it is threatening because it means that things may get worse.

To the hopeful it is encouraging because things may get better.

To the confident it is inspiring because the challenge exists to make things better.

King Whitney Jr.

38. Making Things Better

Ruth and Phil's visits impacted me tremendously. I recognized that change needed to occur. I realized that **I** needed to initiate these changes. There were many items that I needed to get done, and I started acting on my hope of changes maybe making things better. Some of the actions that I took included:

- I called the LTFU and asked for help. I simply stated that I wasn't trained or prepared to handle what was going on with the side effects of the Prednisone.
- I called and made a doctor's appointment for myself.
- I made a spreadsheet with every tiny thing I did.
- I put feelers out about needing someone to mow the lawn and help in the garden.
- I wrote sincere thank-you notes to both Ruth and Phil, acknowledging the impact their friendship, honesty, and compassion had on me.

The phone call to the clinic was the start of a renewal of hope for me. We were called to meet with the Red Team, and they began reevaluating Bob. This included blood work, questions, a physical exam, and a meeting with a psychiatrist. Bob had never had any kind of therapy or one-to-one session, so the fact they convinced him to participate was amazing.

His Prednisone was cut back a little, and appointments were made for checkups on a regular basis. I learned that Bob was going to be on the Prednisone for a long time. It was my hope that decreasing Bob's amount of Prednisone, even a small amount, would impact his behavior and attitude. I knew his GVHD was the priority, and he would have to be watched very carefully. The team ordered tests to see if the GVHD was in his gut, maybe causing the diarrhea. I left the clinic not feeling quite as alone. My observations and feelings had been validated. Maybe I wasn't losing my mind. On the drive home I had a surge of calmness and new hope come over me. I knew I had help dealing with and caring for Bob.

I did not have a doctor, so I used the name of someone that one of the other caregivers in the Caregiver Class had recommended. The appointment triggered me to make a list of concerns about my own health. On the top of my list was the pain I had in my right leg with my varicose veins. I had my veins stripped about twenty years prior and the bubbles and pain had all returned. As we talked of my history and pain, the doctor worked on the computer and ordered an appointment with a specialist.

The next item was my sciatic nerve on my right side. It was extremely painful and something that had started acting up during Bob's transplant. I decided to make an appointment with a massage therapist. It was something new for me, and I was open to try anything. My next concern was my anxiety and isolation. The doctor suggested a therapist that would work on a payment plan with me. She also ordered a low-dose prescription of Lorazepam for me to try. I found myself busy following up with appointments and concentrating on changing my outlook and surroundings. I had a new mission. I just wanted to feel and be healthy.

The spreadsheet I made had two purposes. The first was to see in black and white what I had taken on. The second was to visually show Bob what little he was contributing to the house and me. I was hoping it would produce a change and things might get better. On the list I included feeding Angel, taking Angel out for a walk, loading and unloading the dishwasher, making beds, taking garbage out, preparing the pill box for Bob, doing laundry, weeding, watering plants, paying bills, mowing, and even attending to the moles. At the top of the spreadsheet I had the dates, and on the first day I just left the printout on the counter. With a red pen I started putting my initial, C, next to each item I did throughout the day.

The next day Bob got up before me and took Angel out for her morning potty walk and fed her before I got up. I found a big B in black ink next to the items he had done. I had to smile to myself. The list had triggered something in him. Maybe it was his competitive nature coming out. I didn't care why he was doing it. I recognized it as change. This was a good thing.

As the days passed, Bob continued to add more and more black Bs next to items on the sheet. He was challenged, and it was a game. I was in seventh heaven. I was getting help with chores, and he was up out of his chair doing things for a change. The interest in the spreadsheet lasted a little over two weeks. The change inspired me to believe in the possibility that things were getting better.

My garden angel came to me through my neighbor, who asked her gardener if he would mind taking on another job and do the mowing for me. I met with Salvador, and yes, he would do it weekly. He not only mowed but trimmed, weeded, and helped out with even the moles. My knees, veins, and sciatic nerve were forever grateful.

The results of the testing done at the clinic confirmed that Bob had GVHD in his gut. They had tried a process called PUVA to control the GVHD on his skin. It was a UV light treatment. It had helped, but it did not stop the spots from coming. Now they had to come up with a plan for his gut.

The plan turned out to be photopheresis. It was a form of apheresis, in which his blood was treated with photoactive drugs, which were then activated with ultraviolet light. The machine used was rare and expensive, with only a few facilities performing the process. The team felt this process would work from the inside out. A special port was surgically put into Bob's chest, and the procedure began. He started out having it done every other week. The process took two consecutive days, with each visit lasting between four to five hours. A new group of nurses and caregivers became our support system.

In mid-July Bob came down with a severe cough and slight fever. We ended up at the ER with Bob being admitted. After many tests it was concluded that he had an infection in his heart valve. The doctors felt that the port line might be the cause and voted to take the port out. After removing the port, the doctor told Bob that the port line was clean. The port was not the cause of the infection in the heart valve.

Although I had started making some changes and taken some actions, the hospital visit triggered my anger. Whenever I walked into Bob's hospital room, he was demanding and short with me. He would sit in the bed with the television on, playing games on the iPad in his lap, and never acknowledge that I was there.

My visits became shorter and shorter. I would go home and work in the garden or sit in my favorite Adirondack chair and just close my eyes and try to breathe. I tried to reason that he was scared and nervous, but I couldn't let go of the hurt I was carrying around. I had no patience. Even though I had been hopeful that things were going to get better, I found myself lacking the confidence to believe it.

*Every single thing you've been through,
every single moment that you've come through,
were all to prepare you for this moment now.
... Who you are, what you do, begins right now.*

Lisa Nichols
The Secret

39. A New Beginning

Bob healed from his infection and was ready to resume the photopheresis. The team scheduled a surgery date to have his port replaced in his chest. We were back on track, visiting Seattle every other week for the procedure.

During one of Bob's procedure days, I decided to stop in at a shop attached to the apartment that we had lived in for five months during the transplant. This shop was unique in that it had items to accommodate cancer patients. I had purchased several pairs of special stockings for Bob and bought a scarf and cards for myself in the past. I liked supporting them. I was told that they would measure my legs for support stockings and send me home with the perfect fit. The surgeon I had visited for my varicose veins recommended wearing the stockings. I was very familiar with them from twenty years earlier.

As I walked into the shop, I recognized one of the gals I had talked with many times during our stay. She rounded the counter and gave me a big hug. "How are you? How is your husband doing?" she asked me. I updated her and told her why I was there. She directed me to the girl that would help me, and as I was sitting down getting my leg measured she sat down next to me and said, "You know … ." She hesitated as she looked into my eyes and then continued, "If you ever want to talk to someone, I know a marvelous clergyman at the clinic. He is wonderful." I looked up and met her eyes. I knew she understood and recognized a change in me in the year since she had seen me. I smiled and said, "I would really like his name."

I made the appointment with Clergyman Stephen on a day that Bob was having a treatment. I was apprehensive, knowing that it was a new person and really, what could be accomplished in forty-five minutes? In the back of my mind I thought maybe being a member of the clergy, he would approach things differently. He greeted me and led me into a small room and listened to me tell my story in about thirty minutes. He spoke softly and did not interrupt me. When tears came to my eyes, I could see understanding in his.

As I took a breath and stopped talking he started talking. "I hear you say you miss who you were. I think I have your new mantra." I blinked and looked at him. "Really?" I said, "A mantra?" He continued summarizing that he heard me say I missed my caring self. He continued, "I don't think you have lost your compassion, it is still there. That is why I feel your new mantra should be the word compassion." I went quiet. I was thinking about what he had said. I was hopeful that he was right. He continued, "Whenever you are triggered or angry with your husband, repeat your mantra. It will help you remember that he is a patient." I smiled and said I would try it.

That night I couldn't help but go over the conversation in my mind. I went to sleep thinking about it. At four in the morning, Bob got out of bed moaning and running to the bathroom. He had diarrhea, and it followed him from the bed to the bathroom. I hit the floor running. I was in the laundry room putting on rubber gloves, slamming the bucket under the faucet, and getting the cleaning supplies out. I leaned over and stopped moving. I looked up and said out loud, "Compassion." I repeated the mantra as I rounded the corner to begin cleaning the floor. Bob was just coming out of the bathroom and stripping off his pajamas. I started the bathwater and said, "Why don't you soak for a few minutes?"

I was on my hands and knees cleaning and felt my anxiety and anger diminish. It was then that Bob looked over at me and said, "I'm sorry. Thank you for cleaning up." It was the first time I had heard a thank you from him since the transplant. I melted. I felt compassion for him. I knew it was not his fault that he had diarrhea, nor did he want to have it. I realized he wasn't punishing me or hurting me on purpose. This revelation and calmness came from practicing my new mantra. Could this really work? I was anxious to practice it again.

I had many incidents occur where I would repeat the word compassion out loud. Eventually, I would just think it. It was my turning point of not feeling used and unheard. It allowed me to move out of myself and once again practice compassion.

The meeting with Clergyman Stephen took place in August. I had continued to practice my mantra as my anxiety and stress were still triggered. I was extremely stressed over our upcoming trip to Kauai. We had missed our trip during the transplant and had picked October as the time we would try to go again. Bob was still on Prednisone and his behavior was still risky and unsafe at times. My mother would be meeting us there, and I couldn't calm myself that things would be all right.

He would want to snorkel, and he had been warned by the nurses to be careful not to get near the coral. His skin was thin, and infection was still a concern. The biggest warning from the nurses and doctors was the sun exposure. Posttransplant patients are more susceptible to skin cancer. They reminded Bob that he must have sunblock on at all times and even to wear long-sleeved shirts. His attitude was, "Okay, sure." He would do what he wanted to do when he got out of sight.

I approached the trip logically. I needed help while there. I wanted it to be a vacation for me too. I didn't want to be on 24-7 while in paradise. I started calling my siblings and asking them one by one if they would like to vacation with us in Kauai. One by one, they responded with reasons why it wouldn't work out. It was short notice. There were no takers.

My one brother, Charles, had said no because of finances. He was available, but he just couldn't do it. I called him a few days after he said no and told him that it wasn't just an invitation for a vacation.

I explained to him that I needed help with Bob. I needed someone to be able be with him and snorkel, play tennis, and keep him safe. He was surprised and asked, "Why didn't you just tell me from the start what was going on?" I tried to explain that it was hard for me to ask for help. I just told him bluntly that I truly needed help. He accepted my offer to fly him out, and he was my hero on that vacation.

There was one incident early on in the vacation that was a turning point for me. Bob and Charles suited up to go snorkeling, and I walked down to the beach with them to watch and take pictures. I heard myself say to Bob, "Please, be careful and stay away from the coral. Did you put sunblock on? Maybe you should wear a long-sleeved shirt." I was a nervous wreck. I watched the two of them as a mother watches her children. Oh yes, I was in hovering mode.

Bob was the first one to come to shore, and as he walked out of the water I could see blood on his chest. I ran to him with a towel and my mouth spewing words. As I was attending to Bob, I saw Charles approaching us. He had blood dripping from his hand. "That coral is nasty!" he commented. It hit me like a lead balloon. Bob didn't bleed from being reckless. The coral got Charles too, and he was a younger, stronger man than Bob. It just happened. I started smiling as I got it.

We traveled to San Diego for the months of January and February. I scheduled friends and family to visit during the two months. The list represented special people. My sister, Judy, and her husband Jim; Charles and Mom; my friend Sharan and her husband; Ruth; Minda; Tyler, my spinning instructor from years past; Anastasia and her friend Scott; and Robert and his new fiancé, Laura. We had eight days alone during the two months. I realized what it meant to me to have friends and family near me. I felt their love and support, and it brought me joy to share myself with them.

While in San Diego my knee went out, and I was using a cane and, at times, a wheelchair. I visited an orthopedic surgeon and received two separate shots in my knee. I was completely dependent on Bob to walk and care for Angel. He would walk down the hundred steps to the beach and walk Angel on the doggie beach and return up the same steps with no problems. I reflected on how handicapped I was now and he was covering for me. How humbling it was. I accepted the circumstances and thanked Bob daily for all the help he gave.

One day while Mom and Charles were visiting us in San Diego, we stopped at Costco to have the lens put back in my glasses. I took a number at the optical department and glanced around at all the people. My eyes settled on a woman across from me, who was leaning against the wall and looking down at the ground. After about five minutes I wandered over and stood by her and asked what number she was and how long she had been waiting.

Our entire conversation lasted less than five minutes. I inquired if she lived in San Diego or was visiting. She was visiting. We discovered we were both from the Seattle area. I shared with her how we ended up in Seattle for Bob's transplant. "In fact," I said, "I am writing a book about it." I told her we moved from Colorado, and she shared she had a daughter who lived five miles from where we used to live in Colorado. We had both been born in Michigan. As her number was called, she told me she was a publisher and author. She handed me her card and told me to check her out, and when I was ready to go forward with my book to call her. I did just that.

Journey's End

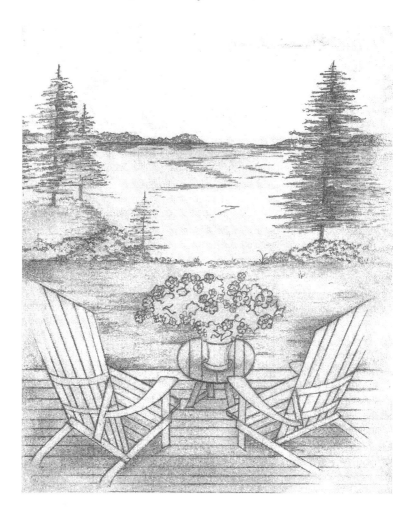

Bob completed his two-year checkup at the clinic and celebrated birthday number two on July 1. He is no longer on Prednisone, and his last immune-suppressing drug has been cut in dosage. His GVHD is calm, with only his eyes being affected. He is weaned from the clinic, and his checkups are with his primary care physician and oncologist.

Today Bob is quite different. Being controlling and needing to be right are no longer parts of his personality. He has softened and compromises daily. The Prednisone Bob has completely disappeared. The bad behavior of a year ago is a thing of the past. He is pleasant with thank-yous often said. He tells me he loves me and compliments me frequently.

We still live on the island of our dreams. My mother at eighty-nine years old has moved in with us. She enjoys the surroundings and the beautiful views with us. We are visiting many of the same wonderful doctors for her health care.

Robert married his soul mate, Laura, and moved from Vancouver, BC, to Boston. It was an event that Bob never dreamed he would live to see. Anastasia is happy and at peace. As parents we are proud of her work ethic and the beautiful woman she is.

I am tired but yet at peace. I still retreat to my favorite quiet place on the deck. I have pronounced this year as MY year. I am determined to address my health issues. My immediate concerns are my knees and pain from the sciatic nerve. I am committed to exercise, eating healthy, and sharing the workload with others. I am scheduled for knee-replacement surgery in a few months.

My approach to each day is much calmer. I find myself not looking or worrying about the future like I used to. Deep down I know that things could change in an instant, but the difference is that I also know that I will be able to handle whatever comes my way. My inner security, strength, and hope are renewed daily by faith, friends, family, and LOVE.

I wish you the same in your journey.